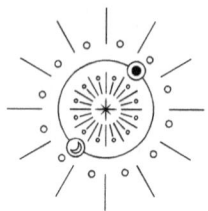

Dedicated to
MJ - Thank you for all your help
and support and for our amazing hive mind.
For always my soul sister.
Cugs

Teanna

www.TeannaTaylor.com

© Teanna Taylor 2025 All Rights Reserved

First Edition 2025
TMJ Publishing
ISBN 978-1-917816-03-8

Copyright & Disclaimer
No part of this publication may be copied, reproduced, stored, or transmitted in any form or by any means - electronic, mechanical, photocopying, recording, or otherwise - without the prior written permission of the copyright owner and publisher.
This book is intended for informational and educational purposes only. It is not intended as, nor should it be considered a substitute for, professional medical advice, diagnosis, or treatment. Always consult with your physician or another qualified healthcare provider regarding any medical condition or health-related concerns. Never disregard professional medical advice or delay seeking it because of THE information contained in this publication.
While every effort has been made to ensure the accuracy and usefulness of the content, neither the author nor the publisher accepts any responsibility or liability for any loss, harm, or damage - whether direct or indirect - that may result from the use or misuse of the information provided herein.

Unlock your
Cosmic Flow

Manifest Your Dreams in Harmony
with Nature's Rhythms

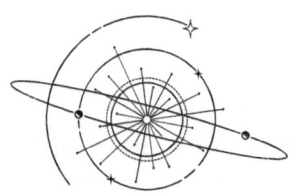

Teanna Taylor

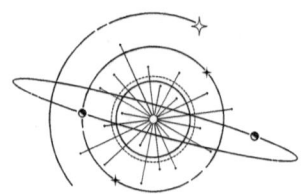

Contents

Letter..5
Dark Days..8
Why Cosmos And Not Universe 14
Children Of The Cosmos................................16
The Science of Cosmic Flow?........................20
Cosmic Confusion 30
Why Are We Out Of Sync 38
How Dates Affect Us 42
Training Your Brain 48
Meditation And The Brain 56
Brain and Heart Coherence 66
Manifesting With Cosmic Flow.......................69
How Long Does It Take To Manifest 71
The 6 Steps to Manifesting with Cosmic Flow ...74
1 Aligning With Cosmic Energy 76
    Spring 77
    Summer 79
    Autumn 81
    Winter 83
2 Review and Reflect 86
    The Ikigai 87
    Life Balance Wheel 94
3 Set Your Intentions 98
4 Emotional Connection 100
    Visualisations..104
    Journaling and Scripting........................108
    Embodiment...110
    Sound and Movement............................112
    Affirmations...114
    Gratitude..122
    Meditation Techniques..........................124

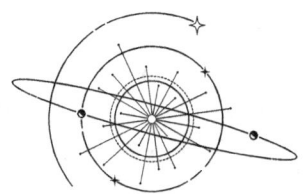

Contents

Cosmic Flow Meditation - Walk through 128
   Recorded Mediation can be found on line
5 Trust and Flow 132
   Synchronicities, Opportunities And Intuition 134
6 Inspired Action 136
Putting It All Together 140
   Daily Routine for Spring 142
   Daily Routine for Summer 144
   Daily Routine for Autumn 146
   Daily Routine for Winter 148
Real Life Examples 150
Cosmic Flow as a Way of Life 152
Feeling Cosmic Energy 158
Overcoming Challenges 162
Limiting Beliefs..164
Empowering Beliefs...168
Personal Affirmations..172
SCAN..188
Conclusion...190

Reference Guides 193
   New Year Resolutions Vs Manifestations..................195
   Setting Intentions...199
   Learning Style Quiz 209
   Meditation and Chakras 213
   Sound Frequencies 217
   Frequencies of Numbers 221
   Shadow Work 227
   Dream Work 231
   Pomodoro Technique 234
   Inner Critic Vs Inner Coach 237
   How to Hack Your Brain 241
   Quick Fixes To Overcome Emotional Challenges....261

Hi Cosmic Explorer

Our paths have crossed for a reason, and only time will tell what that is, but I intend to hold space for you as you continue on your journey called life, a space of time which I hope will be the beginning of an incredible journey towards your dream life of fulfilment and contentment. I have taught these exercises in small groups and one-on-one, as people have crossed my path for a long while now, and it is these groups that have encouraged me to write them down in a book so that I may help many more.

My journey is a long, hard one, one I would not wish on anyone, but from it, I have learnt a lot, experienced some profound moments, gained clarity, and learnt to flow. I touch on my journey in the first chapter. But you have found this book for you. And although my experience is essential; the words here allow you to learn something about yourself, and I hope you ultimately 'trust and flow' too.

The book's first part covers Cosmic Flow principles, followed by the practical steps and tools you can use to manifest, within time you will not need these – as you will just flow – but they will help you on your journey. The last part of the book contains reference guides, which I have included to help you overcome the elements that make us human so you may feel the flow more quickly. I have also created four workbooks, which hold your hand through the seasons and encourage you to work with the energy of that season. As I mentioned before, in time, you will flow as you feel the energy naturally.

I know understanding Cosmic Flow can sound complicated, but it is straightforward. It is about surrendering and overcoming the limiting beliefs you have formed on your journey and becoming aware of energy and the synchronicities around you.

It is not just 'understanding' that at our core, we are energy – experiencing life through our thoughts, emotions, and actions – but 'accepting' that we are just energy, here to experience life. And when we die, we remain as energy.

Energy is nothing new; it was there at the dawn of time, it is in fact, what everything is – just energy – but its flow is something many have lost touch with – it is a bit of a paradox in that we as humans have asked the question of 'why' and quantum physics is beginning to answer – but on that collective journey we have forgotten the 'how'. I am not surprised; getting lost in the hustle is easy, and we are distracted by the technology around us daily. But this disconnection can be frustrating, especially when you sense something deeper is at play. Perhaps you've doubted your worthiness in pursuing your dreams or felt pressure to conform to external expectations. These limiting beliefs can create resistance, blocking the natural flow of energy in our lives. But here is the good news: You are not stuck. This book is designed to help you recognise and release these barriers, offering practical techniques to realign with your authentic self, find your soul purpose and reconnect with the energy of the Cosmos.

As we explore these spiritual and energetic principles, I will also integrate insights from neurology, psychology, and quantum physics – disciplines that bridge the mystical with the scientific. These fields offer valuable perspectives on the nature of reality and consciousness and how our thoughts, emotions and actions shape our experiences. Understanding this balance can help us navigate life's challenges with greater awareness, resilience, and grace.

It is completely natural if you approach these ideas with scepticism or uncertainty. Questioning is an essential part of growth. Together, we will explore these concepts with curiosity, openness, and compassion, allowing space for clarity to emerge in your own time.

Ultimately, I hope to support you in rediscovering your connection to Cosmic energy, helping you cultivate clarity, balance, and a more profound sense of belonging. Whether you seek personal growth, healing, or simply a greater understanding of ease in life, remember that you are not alone. The Cosmic Energy guides you gently, patiently, and with infinite wisdom.

Let's take this journey together. Let's embrace the flow.

Teanna

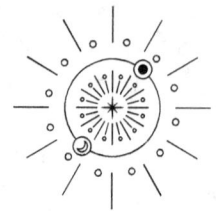

"Even in the dark there is tenacity!"

Teanna

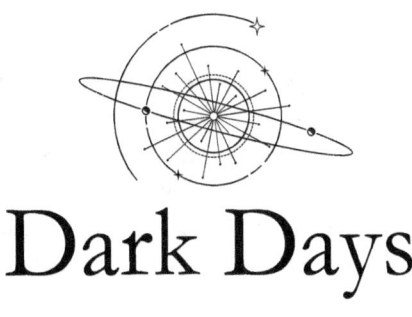

Dark Days

From the moment I was born, I carried natural high-vibrational energy, strong empathic instincts, and a deep spiritual awareness. However, these gifts were never nurtured as a child, and for years, I suppressed them until they knocked me for six at age 35. That was the last time I ignored my intuition.

I was pregnant with twins, nearly full-term, and both babies were in a breech position. The doctors advised a Cesarean section, warning me that attempting a natural birth could result in brain damage for the girls. Every cell in my body was screaming at me not to go through with it - I was physically shaking and sobbing, a vibration I had not felt before - every ounce of my being was saying 'no' - but fear won. I felt pressured, conflicted, and powerless. I decided to proceed with the C-section, one I instinctively knew was wrong. Thankfully, my daughters were born healthy, but that moment changed my life forever.

Shortly after the operation, I suffered a severe haemorrhage and experienced what I now recognise as an out-of-body experience. My body was floating in what felt like a warm bath of honey; I then became weightless and free from pain. I watched the nurses from above rush around me, yet I felt no fear - only complete peace and stillness. When I returned to my body, I had no idea it would be the last time I would be pain-free for over a decade.

Following the haemorrhage, I suffered what was initially thought to be a minor stroke (TIA), but it is now believed to have been something far more significant. The lack of oxygen to my brain caused damage and triggered a chronic hemiplegic migraine that persisted 24/7 for six years, followed by another ten years of chronic pain. Yes, it was a migraine that lasted continuously for over six years! And then only brief breaks for another 10 years!

This was more than just a headache. I lost cognitive function, struggled with chronic fatigue, and was unable to process thoughts clearly. My vision, balance, coordination, and memory were severely impaired. Simple tasks, like walking upstairs, reading a book or watching a film, became impossible. My senses were overloaded with sounds, lights, smells, and even touch, which were overwhelming. I lived in near-total isolation, with white walls repainted in soft cream because pure white physically hurt my eyes. There were days I could barely leave my bed, let alone function as the mother I wanted to be.

I experienced ice-pick headaches so intense they knocked me to the floor, vertigo, Alice in Wonderland Syndrome, depersonalisation, and even blackouts just from standing up. I could not engage in everyday life, I could not drive, and for long periods, I even struggled to swallow without choking. The world as I knew it fell apart, and I only wanted to regain an essential quality of life. All hopes and dreams had gone.

Despite my suffering, I held onto one unwavering belief: I would beat this, whatever "this" was.

In those years of forced stillness, something incredible happened. Alone in the dark, I learned to listen deeply, surrender to the whispers of intuition, and feel the energy of the frequencies around me. This was where my true awakening began. Advised by a doctor, I turned to meditation, not as an escape but as a lifeline. Over time, I discovered that by tapping into my subconscious and cosmic frequencies, I could begin to reroute my brain, restore my nervous system, and reclaim my energy flow.

What followed was not a quick fix. It took another ten years to say I had 99% normal brain function again. But every step of that journey led me to the most profound truth of my being - meditation is not just something I practice; it is my soul's purpose.

Through my experience, I have studied the science of the brain, the power of energy flow, and the intersection between neurology, psychology, quantum physics, and spirituality. I now dedicate my life to helping others shortcut the journey I endured, using cosmic energy, meditation, and aligned action to create transformation without suffering.

Dark Days

We all experience trauma in different ways, but it does not have to define us. The key is not to ask, "Why did this happen to me?" but rather, "Why did this happen for me?" When we learn to align with the natural flow of the Cosmos, we stop fighting life and start co-creating it. I now know I have Ehlers-Danlos Syndrome[1] I could have given birth naturally (and I discovered that by following the energy vibrations), but at that time, the C-section was the decision I made - the one I knew, to my core, was the wrong one.

I have, of course, pondered that decision a lot and had many tearful moments, especially before I trusted my awareness fully. Interestingly, all my moments of regret have been for the children - our house was often quiet. I was often in bed, although I tried my hardest to be awake when they were about. I used to get up to help prepare them for school, then went straight back to bed and got up just before they came home to spend time with them. We ate together every night, and I was always present at bath time and bedtime, including a short book. Then I went back to bed when they did. That was my life for years - sleep, kids, pain, heal, sleep, kids, heal, pain...

They knew when the migraine was too much for me to bear and instinctively were quiet. I could not play any game which required moving about or needed lots of energy, but we did lots of creative activities (mess makes memories). I would fall asleep watching a movie every time and could not stay on outings for long. My first holiday with them was a week for my 40th birthday, five years after the event, where I spent three days in bed just from the process of actually travelling, so Disney never happened; I could not be a big part of their school life, and PTA would not be for me. I could not provide for after-school clubs, but when you ask them, childhood was full of love, fun, and care, and I was often told, 'You are not like other mums,' by them and their friends. I was present for them; they were well-fed and well-groomed, and we enjoyed every ounce of fun I could master. We honestly smelled roses and watched rainbows. My only regret is that I cannot remember the girls' first steps and only know their first words as it is written down. Thankfully, my now ex-husband was an avid photographer, so I have lots of photos to look back on.

Would I make the same decision again?

---

(1) Ehlers-Danlos Syndrome (EDS) is a group of inherited connective tissue disorders characterised by hypermobile joints, fragile skin, and abnormal wound healing, caused by defects in collagen production, with symptoms ranging from mild joint instability to severe complications affecting blood vessels and internal organs.

Of course not. I would listen with my whole being now and trust my feelings. Do I feel regret? No, I have come to terms with it and understand that everything happens for a reason. That one decision changed my life forever. A minor stroke and a ten-year migraine were never on any plan, but without going through what I did, I would not know what I know now, and that includes not ignoring that strong frequency again - everything is for a reason.

The journey took me down two simultaneous yet very separate paths - one of chronic illness and migraine advocacy and the other of spiritual awakening. I knew these would come together one day, but I did not know how until I started to write this.

During quiet hours alone in a dark room, of which there were thousands, I learnt to appreciate the small things, listen to the whispers of my intuition, and feel the energy of the frequencies around me. And most of all, I learnt to meditate! There is enough material from this journey to fill a book on its own, but this book is not about me; this one is about you and some of the lessons I learnt along the way, as I knew one thing for sure: deep inside my soul, that one day I would prevail. I never faulted on that belief. It is one of the reasons that I am here today to tell the tale and stand as a testament to the fact that working with Cosmic frequencies works. I rerouted my brain and brought the faulty internal natural systems back online. I have learnt a lot about Cosmic energy, the power of meditation, how the brain functions, spiritual awakening and how it links to science.

I am writing this today with the vision of helping those stuck with any human-based issue, circumventing the journey I had to go through and 'hacking' the system per se. Teach not just about the frequencies within and around us but also to go deeper and feel the frequencies of Cosmic flow and align with them.

Life is for living, and we all experience trauma in some shape or form. Still, we should be able to experience human existence in such a way that the trauma, drama, illness, and limiting beliefs we hold come into balance. We should grow from them and balance them in order to let their hold over us go.

You found this book and the workbooks for a reason - that reason is deep down in your soul, calling you to make changes - to empower yourself, love yourself and move on in life in a more connected, contented, balanced way, full of abundance and joy in your heart. I look forward to holding your hand as you take the first steps.

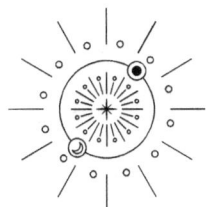

"The human spirit is stronger than anything that can happen to it."

C.C. Scott

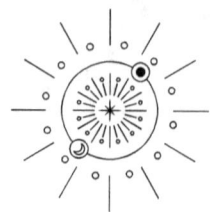

*"The
Universe
is a thing,
the
Cosmos
is everything"*

Teanna ♡

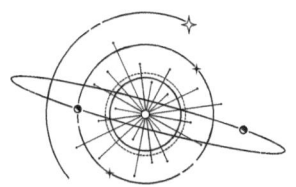

Why Cosmos and Not Universe?

Whilst 'Universe' and 'Cosmos' are often used interchangeably, they have slightly different meanings regarding energy flow.

In scientific terms, the 'Universe' represents the observable reality and everything contained within it - the totality of all space, time, matter, and energy that currently physically exists. It includes everything from the smallest particles to the largest galaxies, the physical laws governing them, and all the stars and planets.

On the other hand, the term 'Cosmos' derived from the Greek word Kosmos, meaning 'order' or 'arrangement' refers not only to the physical realm but also the energetic ones, and the idea of an ordered, harmonious system that connects all things, past, present and future, so the 'Cosmos' does not just refer to the material world, but to the deeper understanding that everything has a place and purpose within the greater scheme of things on an energy level.

It emphasises the interconnectedness of all things and the underlying harmonies, including things we do not even know about yet - multiverses are already theoretically possible within our understanding of physics - so the Cosmos would incorporate all of these, too. It also includes all states of energy frequencies, including our changing frequency cycles from living to dead to living.

Even though everything is energy, everything presents differently depending on its vibration. All these different representations have to ebb and flow together. When in sync, they are a beautiful rhythm of contentment and flow, but when out of sync, they feel very off and stagnant and can cause illness. This is why manifestation is often seen as something challenging to work with.

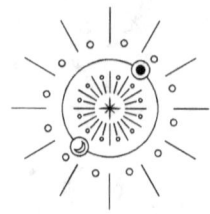

*"Everything is made
up of energy,
and by understanding
and
working with it,
we can enhance
our spiritual,
emotional,
and physical lives"*

Teanna

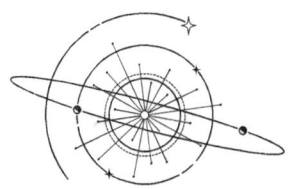

Children of the Cosmos

*"We are all energy -
all children of the Cosmos"*

Teanna

At the heart of Cosmic Flow is the notion of unity - the understanding that a vibrational frequency of energy interconnects everything. This invisible field of energy and information exists beyond time and space, connecting everything in the Cosmos. Our thoughts and emotions interact naturally with this energy flow, shaping our reality daily.

Like our breath, which keeps us alive, Cosmic Energy Flow works daily, automatically humming in the background and shaping our reality. However, at this stage, it may be something you are unaware of or feel out of your control. But, once you bring your awareness and align to this energy flow, you can influence your experiences and overall well-being. Just like when you become aware of your breath, whilst it is still working for you 24/7, you can still control it once you bring your awareness to it.

Different traditions and philosophies describe this energy in various ways; for example, in Taoism and Traditional Chinese Medicine (TCM), this energy is called Qi (Chi), while in Hinduism and Yoga, it is referred to as Prana. In Japanese Reiki, it is called Ki. In science, this is called the Quantum Field.

Whatever the various traditions call it, it is all the same - 'Energy from the Cosmos'. When we align with its flow, we develop a deeper connection to ourselves and our surroundings, fostering a sense of ease and unity. We naturally do this without thinking, just as we breathe without thinking.

The flow responds, even if we are not aware of it. It responds not to what we 'want' but to 'how we feel.' If we feel stress, fear or uselessness, we attract more of the same, whereas if we cultivate gratitude, joy, and love, we align with new possibilities.

By repeatedly feeling the same way, we reinforce the same life circumstances and can get ourselves into cycles without being conscious of them - positive or negative. But by shifting our internal state, we can create a new external reality. And yes, we all have control over this.

Through deep meditation, we can detach from our identity, access a natural flow, and reprogram our subconscious mind for transformation. This process includes healing, self-development, and manifestation. The keys, however, are not to want but to feel and not focus on all the fine details, especially concerning how things will happen.

For example, when we become aware of our breathing, we naturally take a deep breath, as we instinctively know that we need more oxygen in our bloodstream. But we breathe in, trusting that the oxygen will enter our bloodstream. We do not concern ourselves with the intricate details of how the oxygen will break down in our cells, go through our lungs and heart, etc. (Did you take a deep breath while reading that paragraph? That was because you became aware of your breathing - see how this works?)

Similarly, when working with Cosmic Energy, instead of fixating on how something will manifest:

> *"We must trust the intelligence of the flow, allowing reality to unfold in unpredictable ways".*

Teanna

This creates a natural flow where circumstances align seamlessly, enabling us to experience peace, balance and harmony. We become more aware of our intuitions and synchronicities, and manifestation becomes effortless as we align with our life purpose.

So, manifestation is not about forcing things to happen; it is about tuning into an elevated state of self-development where our energy aligns with our desired future. I refer to this as aligning with "The Frequencies of Cosmic Flow." And we can alter our frequency by changing our vibration through gratitude, meditation, and positive action. By doing so, we maintain a balance that fosters health and spiritual harmony, allowing us to attract what we truly need. Additionally, we can heal physical, mental and emotional issues. I certainly did!

To connect with the Cosmic Flow, I recommend daily meditation, generating elevated emotions, visualising desired outcomes, letting go of attachment to the results and trusting that the flow will organise events in alignment with our state of being. This concept challenges traditional views of pure fate and determination, emphasising that we are not victims of our past but creators of our reality. Through conscious intention and emotional alignment, anyone can heal by physically changing the neurological pathways, manifesting abundance, and embracing a new personal reality via neuroplasticity.

Therefore, instead of resisting life's inevitable changes, Cosmic Flow embodies "Trust and Flow." This is a state of letting go of controlling outcomes and setting solid goals, relinquishing rigid expectations.

This encourages us to embrace the unfolding of events, believing that everything occurs for a reason and serves a purpose.

Just like oxygen, Cosmic Energy Flow is fundamental to our existence. By becoming aware of and working with it, we can achieve more than inner peace, balance and spiritual growth.

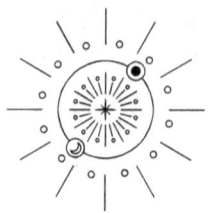

"Setting an intention is planting a seed in the Cosmos - nurture it with belief, and watch your reality bloom."

Teanna

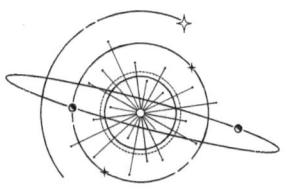

The Science of Cosmic Flow

Cosmic flow is the idea that the universe moves in a natural, intelligent rhythm and that when we align ourselves with that rhythm, life tends to unfold with more ease, clarity, and meaning. It is not about control or hustle. It is about recognising that we are part of something bigger, and choosing to move with it, rather than against it.

You can think of cosmic flow like a river. When you are in the current, things move, you are supported, decisions feel clearer, and opportunities show up. There is a kind of grace to everything. But when you resist - when you try to swim upstream because of fear, pressure, or control - you often feel stuck, anxious, or burnt out. The effort is immense, and progress feels slow.

So, what does it mean to actually be in flow with the cosmos? It means paying attention, listening to your inner wisdom, trusting in timing, and noticing when life opens up and when it contracts. It is about being aware of patterns, energy shifts, and even synchronicities - those little "coincidences" that are not coincidences at all.

I want to be clear: cosmic flow does not mean life becomes perfect or challenge-free. It means that you start working with life, not fighting it. You begin to recognise that everything has a season, and just like the moon waxes and wanes, so do we. There are times to act and, times to rest, times to plant, and times to wait. The more you honour that, the less resistance you feel - and the more aligned your actions become.

Practices like meditation, journaling, breathwork, and even spending time in nature are all tools that help us tune in. They quiet the noise so we can actually hear what life is asking of us. And when we move into that place, we are not just reacting - we are co-creating.

So the next time you feel stuck or like you are pushing too hard, ask yourself: Am I in flow? Or am I forcing something that is not ready? Chances are, the cosmos is not blocking you - it is guiding you. And the more you learn to listen, the more you realise that you are not separate from the cosmos. You are it. You are made of the same stars, breath, and pulse.

When you remember that and move with that truth, that is cosmic flow.

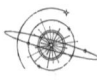 ## Quantum Physics

Everything in our world is made up of energy, from the air we breathe to the water we drink and the mobile devices we use. They just vibrate at different frequencies.

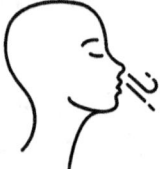 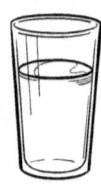 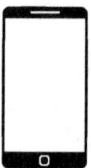

All made up of the same thing

The first dissection level is Atoms, which consists of a central nucleus comprising subatomic particles (which means it is unbelievably tiny). These are called protons and neutrons. This nucleus is surrounded by an electron cloud where electrons are likely to be found. I have drawn the diagram below showing the nucleus much larger than it actually is, as I do not have a big enough piece of paper! The electron cloud can be up to 100,000 times larger than the nucleus.

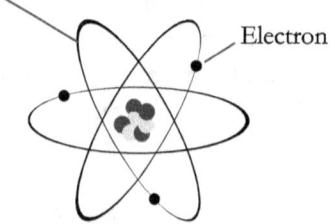

Nucleus - composed of Protons and Neutrons

Although atoms may have different appearances, they are fundamentally composed of identical subatomic particles, i.e. protons, neutrons, and electrons. However, not all atoms are identical; they vary in type, known as 'elements,' each with distinct physical and chemical properties. You may have heard of some of these elements, such as oxygen, carbon, and gold, but not others, like bismuth, xenon, and osmium. But they all appear on the periodic table, which organises these elements by atomic number, which is determined by the number of protons in the nucleus.

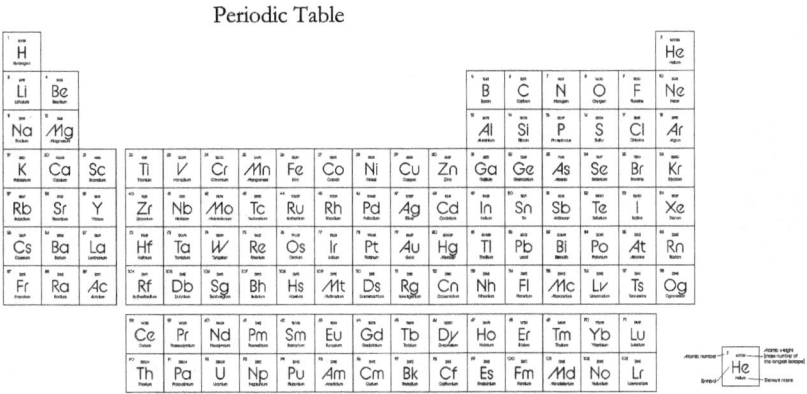

Periodic Table

Quantum physics is a fascinating branch of science that deals with the behaviour of matter and energy at the smallest scales, such as atoms and subatomic particles. It challenges our everyday understanding of the world's workings because it follows the rules very different from classical physics.

For example, 'Wave-Particle Duality' shows that electrons and photons (light particles) can behave both as particles and as waves and 'Superposition' is the quantum phenomenon where a single particle exists in multiple states simultaneously until measured. Then there is 'Entanglement', where two particles become linked so that the state of one instantly affects the other, regardless of the distance separating them.

Einstein described this as "spooky action at a distance," but it remains just as mysterious as it sounds!

Examples of matter in different states

Gas
i.e. Oxygen (O_2)
in the air that we breathe.

Liquid
i.e. Water (H_2O)
in a river, ocean, or a glass.

Solid
i.e. A rock, metal, or a wooden table.

Plasma
i.e. the Sun, lightning, or a neon sign.

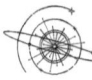 ## Matter from Molecule to Quark

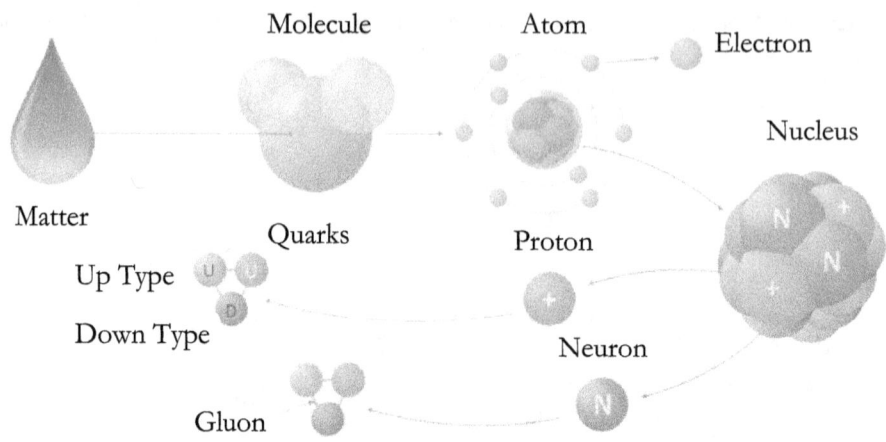

This was proven over a longer distance in 2017 by researchers at the University of Vienna and the Austrian Academy of Sciences, who conducted an experiment demonstrating quantum entanglement between the Canary Islands of La Palma and Tenerife, a distance of 144 kilometres. They used a powerful laser to send unique light particles called photons from one island to another. These photons were entangled, which means they were connected in a strange, invisible way. Whatever happened to one photon also happened to the other, even though they were far apart. This experiment showed that these particles stay connected no matter how far apart they are. It was like they were communicating instantly, faster than the speed of light! This was a big step toward creating super-fast and super-secure quantum communication networks in the future.

The exciting thing about quantum physics is that it is not just theoretical; it is the foundation for many modern technologies we rely on today, including semiconductors, lasers, and even quantum computers! Moreover, it challenges our understanding of reality, making it one of the most exhilarating fields of science.

In simple terms, quantum physics helps us understand the composition of atoms - protons, neutrons, and electrons. It explains how these tiny particles interact and form the building blocks of everything around us.

So, the next time you stand outside at night, look around, and gaze at the stars, remember that everything in the Cosmos is fundamentally made of the same thing - including you - you are just the same as the stars!

If you want to explore Quantum Physics more, I recommend the lecture ' A Brief History of Quantum Mechanics' by Prof Sean Carroll at the Royal Institute in 2020. This can be found on YouTube or my website. In this talk, Prof Carroll walks you through the history of quantum discoveries, from Einstein and Bohr to the present day, explaining his favourite theories along the way.

Prof Carroll is a theoretical physicist, specialising in quantum mechanics, gravitation, cosmology, statistical mechanics, and foundations of physics, with occasional dabblings elsewhere. His official titles are Research Professor of Physics at Caltech and Research Professor at the Santa Fe Institute. He has also written a book about this called "Something Deeply Hidden"

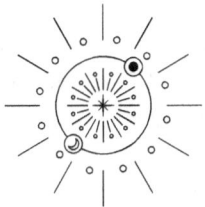

"If quantum mechanics hasn't profoundly shocked you, you haven't understood it yet"

Niels Bohr, a pioneer of quantum mechanics

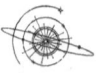 ## Electromagnetic fields

Electromagnetic fields, often abbreviated as EMFs, are invisible areas of energy that surround any object with electrical charge. They are created whenever electricity flows, meaning they are constantly present in our environment. An EMF consists of two parts: electric and magnetic fields. These two forces travel together in waves, and the strength and frequency of those waves vary depending on the source.

EMFs occur both naturally and through human-made technology. Natural sources include the Earth's magnetic field, the sun's radiation, and even the human body - our brain and heart generate tiny electromagnetic fields that can be measured with special equipment. On the other hand, artificial EMFs are produced by mobile phones, Wi-Fi routers, microwave ovens, power lines, and electrical appliances. These modern technologies emit EMFs constantly, especially in urban areas where digital devices are everywhere.

Not all EMFs are the same. They exist on a spectrum that ranges from low-frequency, low-energy fields to high-frequency, high-energy radiation. The lower end includes radio waves and the electricity that powers your home. The higher end includes ultraviolet light, X-rays, and gamma rays, which can harm the body in high doses. Most everyday electronics emit non-ionising radiation, which is generally considered safe in small amounts, though long-term exposure is a growing area of research and debate.

Understanding EMFs matters because they are deeply woven into how the cosmos and our bodies function. The human nervous system, for example, communicates through electrical impulses. Our hearts emit measurable electromagnetic waves that can be detected several feet away. Some scientists and holistic practitioners believe that excessive exposure to artificial EMFs may affect our health, potentially influencing sleep, stress levels, and emotional regulation - especially if we are not balancing that exposure with time in natural environments.

In everyday terms, EMFs are simply the invisible energetic fabric that connects and powers everything - from smartphones to stars to our bodies. Becoming more aware of these fields can help us understand how we interact with technology and the natural world. It also opens the door to more mindful living - choosing when to engage with digital devices, when to disconnect, and how to maintain our energetic balance.

Now, here is where this links to cosmic flow.

At its core, cosmic flow is the idea that everything in the Cosmos - including us - is part of one big interconnected energetic system. We are not just bodies - we are also fields of energy. Our hearts emit electromagnetic waves, our brains emit frequencies, and even our emotions and thoughts carry energetic signatures. So, we are constantly exchanging energy with the world around us, whether we realise it or not.

When we are in a state of calm, presence, gratitude, or love, our energy field becomes more coherent - more balanced, more harmonious. That coherence helps us "tune in" to the greater field of life: cosmic flow. Ideas flow more easily, we feel more connected, and we begin to experience synchronicities - those little signs that things are falling into place.

But when we are stressed, scattered, or constantly bombarded by artificial EMFs - like overstimulation from technology or a high-stress environment - our energy field can become chaotic or depleted. We lose our signal, so to speak. It is like trying to tune into a radio station but getting static. That is when we feel off, disconnected, or out of flow.

This is why practices like meditation, grounding, breath work, time in nature, and digital detoxing are so powerful. They help clear the noise and restore our natural energetic balance. They strengthen our connection to the Earth's electromagnetic field - which is incredibly stabilising - and they help us re-align with the deeper rhythms of life, what we call cosmic flow.

So, in essence, you are a field within a field. Your ability to harmonise with the energy around you - the Earth, other people, or the Cosmos - directly affects how you can hear, feel, and follow that flow.

When your field is aligned, your life is aligned.

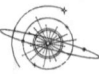 ## EMFs and Wellbeing

While EMFs are a natural part of life, the modern world has amplified our exposure through technology. Our bodies did not evolve to be surrounded 24/7 by artificial electromagnetic frequencies from phones, Wi-Fi, Bluetooth, smart meters, and power lines. For some people, this constant exposure may contribute to symptoms like fatigue, brain fog, irritability, sleep disturbances, and a feeling of being energetically "off." Although science is still exploring the long-term effects of EMF exposure, many people find that reducing digital overload and reconnecting with nature makes a noticeable difference in how they feel.

EMFs, especially artificial ones, can disrupt the body's natural rhythms - like our circadian rhythm (our internal clock), melatonin production (which affects sleep), and our ability to stay grounded and present. When we are overstimulated by tech and disconnected from the Earth, our nervous system can become overloaded, and our energetic field may feel scattered, unprotected, or depleted.

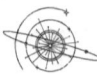 ## Grounding (Earthing)

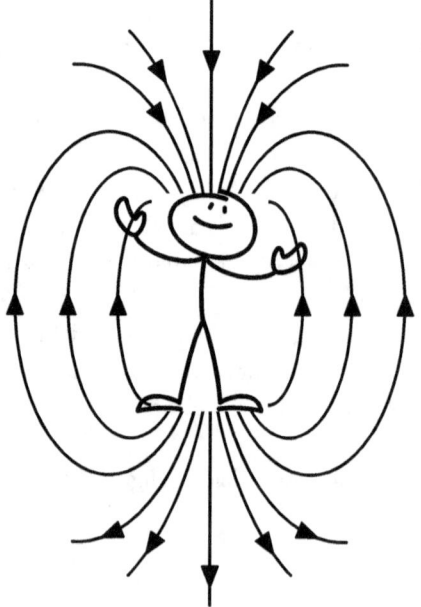

Grounding, also known as earthing, is a simple practice that involves direct physical contact with the Earth - like walking barefoot on grass, sand, or soil. The Earth carries a negative electrical charge, and when we connect to it, we absorb free electrons that help neutralise excess positive charge in our bodies (which can accumulate from EMFs and stress).

Some studies have shown that grounding reduces inflammation, improves sleep, lowers cortisol (the stress hormone), and even regulates heart rate variability. But beyond science, people often describe it as feeling calmer, clearer, and more present - as though their energy is being stabilised and reset. In energetic terms, it is like plugging back into your natural power source.

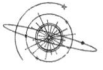 ## Breathwork

Breathwork is another powerful tool for balancing your energy field and nervous system in a world full of EMFs and stimulation. When we constantly absorb energy from screens and environments, our breath often becomes shallow or erratic, which reinforces stress. Conscious breathing - deep, slow, rhythmic - helps regulate the autonomic nervous system, promoting relaxation, mental clarity, and emotional release.

Energetically, in many traditions, breath is a life force - prana or chi. Through intentional breathing, we can clear energetic blockages, increase flow, and return to our coherence. It is a way to reconnect to the natural rhythm within, even when everything around us feels fast, chaotic, or overwhelming.

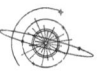 ## Energy Healing

Practices like Reiki, crystal healing, sound therapy, and intuitive energy work all work on the premise that the human body is not just physical but energetic. These practices aim to restore harmony and balance to the energy body - clearing what does not belong, strengthening what is depleted, and tuning us into our natural frequency.

Energy healing can help shield your field from external noise, release stored emotional or energetic residue, and strengthen your sense of personal presence. It benefits people sensitive to EMFs or who feel energetically drained by crowded spaces, electronics, or constant stimulation.

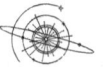 ## Conclusion

Living in a high-tech world does not mean you are doomed to be drained. The key is awareness and balance. When we remember that we are energetic beings living in an energetic world, we can begin to care for ourselves in a more subtle, intentional way. We can use grounding to stabilise, breath work to regulate, and energy practices to clear and recharge.

Ultimately, this is how we return to cosmic flow - not by disconnecting from the world, but by reconnecting with ourselves and the Earth and choosing to live in rhythm with our own energy and the deeper intelligence of life.

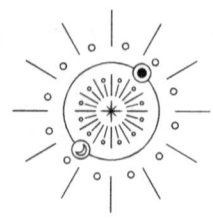

*"We are the children
of the Cosmos,
the offspring of stars,
woven from the fabric of the
universe itself.
The same atoms that burn in
the hearts of galaxies
reside within us,
reminding us that we are not
separate -
we are infinite, we are one"*

Teanna

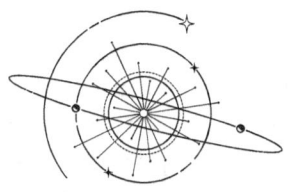

Cosmic Confusion

Just as the tides are influenced by the moon and the seasons by the sun, our energy ebbs and flows in response to these same celestial forces. This should be a natural flow where we feel the energy around us, but over time, we have learnt to ignore these subtle feelings and follow a man-made time structure. Particularly the Gregorian calendar we follow, which is artificial and disregards this connection. It uses fixed months that do not honour the dynamic rhythm of the moon, sun, and seasonal cycles, instead confining us to a rigid structure that distances us from the Cosmic Flow that has guided life for millennia.

The Northern Hemisphere

In January, in the heart of winter, nature slows down. Animals hibernate, and plants lie. Dormant and daylight hours are limited. In this quieter season, our bodies and minds often crave rest, reflection, and planning rather than action or forward momentum.

This disconnection is why many feel stuck, frail, out of sorts, and tired. It is why our January resolutions often fail. Despite the abundance of self-help books, courses, and motivational speeches, something still feels off. We are trying to create miracles at the wrong time. But think about it - would a farmer sow crops in the dead of winter? Of course not. The land is not ready, the seeds would wither, and the effort would be wasted. Yet every January, millions of us engage in this exact folly, setting intentions and goals at a time when both our minds and bodies are craving rest and reflection.

Take a minute and imagine attempting to swim against a raging current - a cold, dark, and angry sea - which is what manifesting in January often feels like. I would like you to envision turning around and allowing the current to carry you forward. Do you feel the energy change? This illustrates the experience of aligning your manifestation practice with the rhythms of the Cosmos - your flow.

Spring is a season of renewal, and psychology shows is the most powerful time to start fresh. As the snow melts, trees bud, and light returns, our brains and bodies naturally begin to wake up from winter's stillness. This environmental shift is not just poetic - it has real effects on our psychology. Subtle cues like more daylight, warmer air, and birdsong activate a sense of possibility, growth, and momentum. We become more energised, optimistic, and ready to take action.

From a biological standpoint, spring gently resets us. The increasing light helps regulate our circadian rhythms, improving sleep, mood, and cognitive function. Unlike the jolt of New Year's resolutions in January - when days are short, energy is low, and our bodies crave rest - spring offers a softer, more sustainable launchpad for change. It is a time when we are more in sync with our biology and more likely to form habits that stick.

Psychologists also point to the "Fresh Start Effect" - people feel more motivated to pursue goals after meaningful transitions or temporal landmarks. Spring is a natural and symbolic fresh start. The world around us is changing, and that sense of external shift often mirrors a desire for internal transformation. Cleaning out the old and making space for something new feels intuitive. Spring cleaning is not just physical - it is psychological.

In contrast, setting resolutions in January, deep in winter, can feel like trying to push a boulder uphill. Nature is dormant, and so are we. Winter is a time of reflection, not reinvention. That is why so many New Year's resolutions fail - not because we are lazy or lack discipline, but because we are trying to force new growth during a season of natural stillness. It is like planting seeds in frozen ground: the intention is there, but the timing is off.

Spring, however, invites us to start slowly and build steadily - just like nature does. Plants do not bloom overnight; they root, sprout, and stretch toward the sun. This mirrors the process of real change: small, consistent steps that grow into something lasting. When we align our personal goals with the season's rhythm, change feels less like a battle and more like a blooming.

So, while the calendar may say the new year starts in January, psychologically and biologically, spring is the true beginning. If we shift our mindset to match the season, we give ourselves a more compassionate and natural starting point that supports us from the inside out.

Season	Northern Hemisphere		Southern Hemisphere	
	Start	Finish	Start	Finish
Spring	Around March 20–21	Around June 20–21	Around September 22–23	Around December 21–22
Summer	Around June 20–21	Around September 22–23	Around December 21–22	Around March 20–21
Autumn	Around September 22–23	Around December 21–22	Around March 20–21	Around June 20–21
Winter	Around December 21–22	Around March 20–21	Around June 20–21	Around September 22–23

These dates can vary slightly year to year depending on the Earth's orbit and leap years.

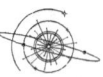

The Southern Hemisphere

January arrives at the height of summer in the Southern Hemisphere. The sun is high, the days are long, and nature is in full bloom. Energy buzzes in the air - plants stretch toward the sky, animals are active, and people gather outdoors. It is a time of warmth, expansion, movement, and celebration.

Oddly, we still follow a global rhythm that tells us January is a time to "start fresh" - to dig deep, set big goals, and kick off new habits. But for us, the true beginning - the natural new year - already happened in spring, back in September, when life was reawakening, the air was fresh with newness, and the earth was soft and ready for seeds of intention.

So what happens in January? We push ourselves to launch into action when, in reality, this is the season for harvesting, celebrating, and simply being. It is not the time to force new beginnings - it is the time to enjoy the fruits of seeds already sown.

No wonder so many of us feel out of sync with January resolutions. It is not that we lack discipline or desire - it is that we are not aligning with the rhythm of the land we live on. We are trying to plant in the summer heat when the soil is full.

So what if we shifted our calendar inwardly - starting our new year in spring when everything is designed to begin again? Growth feels natural rather than forced when the air is charged with potential. What if we let summer and January be a time of gratitude, fullness, and gentle course correction - not pressure?

Nature has wisdom. When we sync with it, we do not have to push so hard - we just have to grow.

Living in the southern hemisphere and making changes is actually easier, as summer energy is not as hard to resist as winter energy. However, spring is still the ideal season to start new resolutions.

Psychology-wise, spring is a season of natural renewal, and our minds and bodies respond to that rhythm. Psychologically, we are wired to feel more hopeful and energised when we notice changes in our environment - flowers blooming, longer days, birdsong returning. These environmental cues subtly signal that it is time to begin again. Researchers have found that even small changes in surroundings can activate context-dependent memory, helping us break free from old habits and create new ones more effectively.

From a neuroscience perspective, spring's gradual increase in sunlight helps regulate circadian rhythms, improve sleep, and boost serotonin levels - all of which will enhance executive functioning (decision-making, planning, self-control). Rather than the high-energy push of summer, spring offers a gentler psychological ramp-up - a better fit for planting the seeds of lasting change rather than forcing rapid action.

Another decisive psychological factor is the "Fresh Start Effect," a well-documented phenomenon where people are more motivated to set and pursue goals after meaningful transition points. Spring is the ultimate fresh start: it marks the end of winter's inward pull and the beginning of outward growth. Unlike January, which in the Southern Hemisphere falls mid-summer and is often full of distractions, spring offers a clean psychological slate with fewer conflicting energies.

Moreover, goal setting in spring is more seasonally aligned with how nature operates. Farmers plant in spring, not summer. Trees begin to bud slowly, not suddenly. Our bodies and minds are also biologically tuned to start new cycles during growth and regeneration. Spring is when we are more likely to feel creative, visionary, and open to forming new routines. Trying to initiate significant changes in summer, when energy is scattered or already at its peak, can lead to over-commitment or burnout - common reasons why resolutions fail.

In summary, while summer may be high-energy, spring is high-potential. It is the season that supports intentional beginnings, thoughtful planting, and gentle momentum. If we align our resolutions with the natural psychology of the season, we are more likely to create habits that do not just spark briefly - but grow, take root, and last.

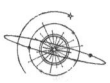 **Equator Alignment**

For those close to the equator, the seasonal patterns we often associate with resolution-setting do not apply similarly - which has a real psychological impact.

For those close to the equator, traditional ideas about seasonal change - like winter giving way to spring - do not quite apply. Near the equator, daylight hours remain relatively constant throughout the year, temperatures are steady, and the year is typically divided into wet and dry seasons rather than the four-season model found in temperate zones. Because of this, people in equatorial regions do not experience the strong external cues - like blossoming trees or snow-covered stillness - that often prompt reflection, rest, or renewal elsewhere.

This lack of dramatic seasonal change impacts how and when people feel naturally inclined to start fresh or set new resolutions. In temperate regions, the transition from winter to spring brings visible change and a psychological sense of possibility. Without those environmental shifts, resolutions near the equator may feel more arbitrary or disconnected from the rhythms of nature. However, this doesn't mean people in equatorial areas are disadvantaged - it just means that different psychological landmarks tend to take precedence.

In these regions, people often respond more to cultural, personal, or social rhythms than environmental ones. The start of a new school year, a birthday, or a significant holiday - like New Year's Day - can act as the internal rhythm.

Equivalent to spring, these events trigger what psychologists call the "Fresh Start Effect," where people feel more motivated to break old habits and start new ones after a clean mental slate. In equatorial climates, the calendar and cultural life become more meaningful anchors for transformation than the seasons themselves.

It is also essential to recognise that, regardless of geography, humans still experience internal seasons - cycles of rest, energy, burnout, renewal, and growth. People close to the equator may not see physical signs of seasonal change, but their minds and bodies still go through emotional and energetic ebbs and flows. Tuning into these personal rhythms - moments of clarity, fatigue, inspiration, or stagnation - can help guide meaningful change more than the natural calendar.

In short, while environmental seasons may not offer strong cues near the equator, the psychology of transformation still applies. People in these regions can benefit from syncing their resolutions with meaningful moments - whether that is the new year or the end of the rainy season.

For many people living near the equator, the end of the wet season and the beginning of the dry season can be an ideal time to set new intentions or begin personal resolutions. While these regions do not experience the classic four seasons, this transition is just as powerful - practically and psychologically. After weeks or months of rain, cloud cover, and often restricted movement, the shift toward drier, clearer days brings a tangible sense of renewal. Much like spring in temperate climates, this time feels like a natural reset.

During the wet season, life can feel slower or more inward-facing. There is often more time spent indoors, disrupted routines, and a general sense of hibernation or waiting. When the rains ease and the dry season begins, people usually feel a rise in energy, optimism, and clarity. The environment becomes more stable and predictable - roads dry up, events resume, and daily life becomes easier to navigate. This external change can mirror an internal one, where people feel emotionally and mentally ready to move forward, make changes, or start fresh projects.

Psychologically, this transition creates the perfect conditions for forming new habits or intentions. The dry season provides consistency, better weather, and more opportunities to be outside, socialise, or work toward goals. This is a crucial foundation for behaviour change - our environment strongly influences our ability to stick with new routines. When the world around us is more supportive, it becomes easier to focus, commit, and grow.

Culturally and symbolically, the end of the wet season often represents a time of emergence. In agricultural communities, this is when the soil has been nourished, and attention turns to growth, maintenance, and preparation for future harvests. This mirrors the human cycle of change: reflection and rest (wet season) followed by action and expansion (dry season). Setting goals at this time aligns with nature's own timeline, making it feel less forced and more grounded.

In summary, while January or the calendar new year may not feel deeply connected for people in equatorial regions, the transition from the wet to the dry season offers a natural, powerful moment to begin again. It marks a psychological shift from inward to outward, from pause to progress. Aligning resolutions with this seasonal rhythm can create deeper motivation, a stronger sense of timing, and a greater chance of meaningful, lasting change.

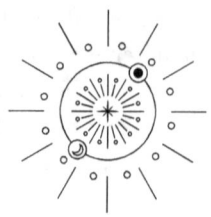

"Nature has already given us the perfect timeline for growth. It whispers to us through the seasons"

Teanna

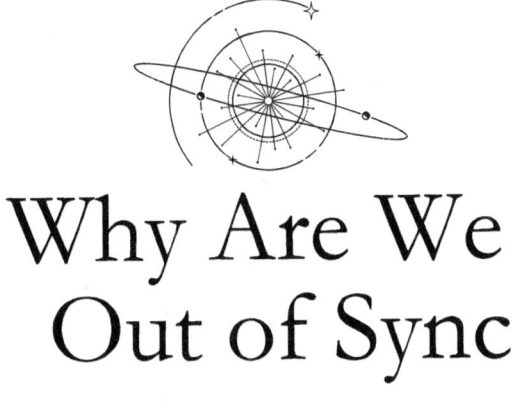

Why Are We Out of Sync

In a nutshell, our man-made calendar, a mix of astronomy, politics, ego, and ancient math, has pushed us out of sync with natural flow.

Today, we use the Gregorian calendar, the world's most widely used civil calendar. But unlike the calculation of 'time', which has been unchanged since 2000 BCE, our calendar has changed significantly over thousands of years.

Its roots are in the Roman Calendar, which is reported, but not proven, to have been created in ~753 BCE by Romulus, the legendary founder of Rome. This calendar had 10 months, starting in March and ending in December, with an unnamed period between the Winter Solstice and Spring Equinox. It was a mix of lunar and solar cycles and poorly structured, which led to seasonal drift over time. This explains why the names are linked to the Roman counting system, i.e., Sep = 7, Oct = 8, Nov = 9, and Dec = 10.

However, the unnamed parts of the calendar were causing problems with agriculture planning, so King Numa Pompilius added January and February in 713 BCE, making it a 12-month calendar. The calendar remained lunar-based but still had flaws, requiring frequent adjustments by priests. At this point, March remained the start of the year.

Within 668 years, the Roman Calendar had drifted out of alignment with the seasons, which again affected agriculture planning. So, in 45 BCE, with the help of Egyptian astrologers, Julius Caesar created the first modern solar calendar based on a 365.25-day year. He introduced the leap year every four years to correct seasonal drift, and for administrative reasons, he declared January 1st as the first day of the year to align with the terms of the new Roman Consuls, who took office on that date.

However, the new calculations slightly overcorrected the shift by 11 minutes and 14 seconds annually, which added up over centuries, causing the calendar to drift 1 day every 128 years.

So, after 1626 years, the calendar had drifted by 10 days, shifting the alignment to the Spring Equinox from March 22nd to March 12th. This was problematic for the Catholic church, as they wanted Easter to be as close to the Spring Equinox as possible, so Pope Gregory XIII corrected this drift, bringing the calendar back in line with the Spring Equinox and Easter calculations. (Easter was officially set as the first Sunday after the first full moon on or after March 21st). He also adjusted the leap year rules, which occur every 4 years, except in centuries not divisible by 400 (e.g., 1700, 1800, and 1900 were not leap years, but 2000 was). He also reaffirmed January 1st as New Year's Day.

In addition to bringing the calendar back in line with the equinox and ensuring the proper timing of religious holidays, a date correction was needed to account for the accumulated 10-day drift. Therefore, the day following October 4, 1582, was declared October 15, 1582.

Catholic countries like Spain, Italy, and France quickly adopted the new system. However, Protestant countries, such as Britain, were hesitant, partly due to the calendar's association with the Catholic Church. As a result, Britain and its colonies, including what would become the United States, did not adopt the Gregorian calendar until another 170 years in 1752. That year, the British Empire skipped 11 days, changing the date from September 2, 1752, to September 14, 1752.

Today, the Gregorian calendar is the standard for most countries, particularly in business, civil matters, and academic settings. As such, it would be challenging to change.

A few countries still use other calendars for specific purposes, such as the Ethiopian or Persian calendars. Some cultures and religions continue to use lunar or lunisolar calendars, such as the Islamic or Chinese calendars.

And in truth, it is just numbers, right?

However, these numbers emphasise a linear progression of days and months, forcing us to adhere to an artificial sense of time.

In contrast, natural cycles (like the seasons and lunar phases) reflect a more circular and holistic understanding of time. Ironically, before the reforms of the Roman Empire, the Christian Church, and the Norman Conquest, Britain used a calendar that aligned with the lunar and agricultural cycles. The Celtic Calendar, often called the Druid Calendar, divided the year into four seasons aligned with critical points in the solar year, such as solstices and equinoxes.

Even in mathematical terms, it makes more sense: It is believed to have had 13 months, with each month corresponding to a moon cycle, the same as women's menstrual cycles. Each month lasted about 28.5 days, which aligns with the moon's synod cycle (the time it takes for the moon to complete an entire cycle of phases). Since 13 months of 28 days (a perfect, regular cycle) would make 364 days a year, this structure would leave an additional day or days to be handled as a special day or festival, often a time of rest or reflection. So, in a nutshell, the Julian and Georgian calendar pushed us out of sync with the natural seasonal flow of the Cosmos.

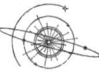

Why 28, 30 and 31 days of the month

The Augustus Twist - There is a rumour (partly true, partly myth) that July (named after Julius Caesar) had 31 days. At the time, August, named after Emperor Augustus, had 30 days. Augustus did not want his month to have fewer days than Julius's, so they stole a day from February and gave it to August!

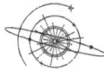

Days of the week

The working week and weekend concept has its roots in a combination of religious tradition, industrial practices, and labour rights movements. The seven-day week dates back to ancient Babylon and was later reinforced by Judeo-Christian beliefs. In the Bible, for example, God is said to have created the world in six days and rested on the seventh, making that day a time for rest and worship. Different religions adopted different holy days: Jews observe Saturday (the Sabbath), Christians observe Sunday, and Muslims hold Friday as a sacred day. This religious influence laid the groundwork for taking at least one day off per week.

However, during the Industrial Revolution in the 18th and 19th centuries, the idea of rest largely disappeared. Factory workers often laboured for six or even seven days a week, with only Sunday typically given off for Christian observance. Many workers - especially those from Jewish communities - pushed for Saturday off as well to align with their religious practices. This pressure influenced factory policies and highlighted the need for more humane working conditions.

In the early 20th century, labour unions became increasingly powerful and advocated for shorter work hours and more time off. One of the most influential moments came in 1926 when Henry Ford implemented a five-day, 40-hour workweek in his factories. This shift was a nod to workers' needs and a move to improve productivity. Ford's model quickly gained popularity, and by 1938, the U.S. government made it official with the Fair Labor Standards Act, which legally established the five-day workweek.

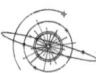 Start to the week

Monday is seen as the first day of the week by most countries; however, psychologically, many studies suggest that Friday tends to be the happiest day for most people, thanks to the anticipation of the weekend and a general sense of relief as the workweek winds down. In terms of productivity, Tuesday often comes out on top. By then, people typically had shaken off Monday sluggishness and were fully engaged in their tasks, making it the most mentally focused day. On the other hand, Monday is widely disliked and seen as the toughest day emotionally, as people struggle to return to routine and face a whole week ahead. Sunday can also be psychologically challenging due to the infamous "Sunday Scaries," when anxiety about the upcoming week starts to creep in - especially in the evening. In contrast, Saturday is considered the most relaxing day, offering the most freedom from work and stress without the looming pressure of the next day.

This is why all my workbooks are designed to begin tasks on Friday - it gives you the best chance to build momentum and set strong intentions. Saturday is then ideal for taking action and physically following through. Starting big goals on a Monday would be unwise, as it is psychologically the most sluggish and mentally unfocused day of the week and one that many people tend to dislike.

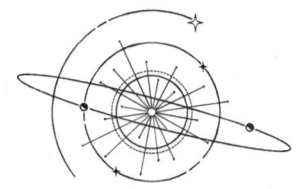

How Dates Affect us

We often hear that "dates are just constructs" and that, technically, you can set intentions and manifest your goals at any time. But the truth is - timing matters. While you can choose to begin again whenever you like, nature's rhythms powerfully influence our bodies and minds. The modern practice of starting the new year in January in the Northern Hemisphere or in September in the Southern Hemisphere is out of sync with the Earth's natural energy flow.

This misalignment shifts the symbolic "new year" away from spring, the true season of renewal, creating tension across every layer of our being. It unnecessarily strains our physical, emotional, mental, and spiritual well-being. Rather than supporting growth, this timing can deplete our energy, cloud our clarity, and make it harder to stay connected to the deeper cycles that govern change. When we push for transformation during seasons meant for rest or recalibration, we disconnect from our natural capacity to thrive.

By returning to nature's beginning anew in spring (around March in the Northern Hemisphere and September in the Southern Hemisphere), we align with the natural momentum of life itself. It is not just about setting goals; it is about co-creating with the energy of the Earth, allowing growth to unfold with more ease, balance, and power.

Body: Disrupting Natural Rhythms and Immunity

Our bodies are guided by the 24-hour circadian rhythm, which is regulated by light and darkness, and longer seasonal rhythms that align with the Earth's natural cycles. These rhythms influence our energy levels, sleep patterns, digestion, immunity, and well-being. When we honour these cycles, we support the body's ability to stay balanced and healthy. But when we go against them - especially in how we set goals and structure our routines - we can create internal stress and resistance.

In the Northern Hemisphere, January arrives in the depth of winter - when the body naturally slows down. Energy is lower, daylight is limited, and the instinct is to rest, reflect, and conserve. It is a season of stillness, not a time to launch into intense changes or high-output routines. Yet, this is precisely when people are encouraged to set New Year's resolutions - often involving strict diets, heavy workouts, or ambitious productivity goals. These demands can clash with the body's natural state, leading to fatigue, sluggishness, low motivation, and burnout.

In the Southern Hemisphere, January falls mid-summer, when energy is high and outward-facing. While this may seem like a natural time to set intentions, it also comes with challenges. The fast pace, heat, social activity, and long days overwhelm the nervous system. For some, this can lead to overexertion, restlessness, or difficulty grounding and focusing on long-term goals. Setting resolutions without attuning to the body's seasonal rhythm in both hemispheres can leave us feeling disconnected, scattered, or emotionally off.

The impacts of forcing change out of sync with the season may include:
- Difficulty maintaining consistency
- Increased self-criticism or guilt
- A sense of being "off" or misaligned
- Goals that fade quickly despite strong intentions

Body: Weakening the Immune System

Seasonal misalignment affects our energy and focus and can strain our immune system. In colder months, especially during winter in the Northern Hemisphere (or winter in the Southern Hemisphere around June–August), the body slows down and conserves energy. Immune function is more vulnerable, metabolism is slower, and our need for nourishment and rest is greater.

Attempting to initiate drastic lifestyle changes during this low-energy period, such as restrictive dieting, intense workout programs, or significant life overhauls, can weaken our immunity rather than strengthen our health. Some common outcomes include:

- **Increased illness**: Pushing too hard in winter can leave us more susceptible to colds, flu, or fatigue-related breakdowns.
- **Slower metabolism**: The body naturally stores more fat and conserves energy in colder seasons, making weight loss efforts frustrating and often unsustainable.
- **Higher inflammation**: Over-stressing the body during its natural downtime can trigger joint pain, exhaustion, and flare-ups in chronic conditions.

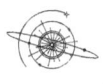 Body: How Seasonal Shifts Affect Eating and Digestion

Our bodies are deeply connected to the cycles of nature, and one of the most immediate ways we feel that connection is through food. We naturally crave different types of nourishment depending on the season-warm, grounding foods in cooler months and lighter, fresher foods in warmer ones. However, modern lifestyles and global wellness trends often ignore these seasonal cues, pushing diets and habits that may be out of sync with our bodies' needs. This can lead to digestive issues, low energy, bloating, and persistent cravings.

In the Northern Hemisphere, January falls in the heart of winter, when the body needs warmth, comfort, and slower digestion. Cold temperatures and shorter days increase cravings for quick energy sources like sweets, carbs, and caffeine. Yet, this is precisely when New Year's resolutions often push cold smoothies, juice cleanses, low-calorie detoxes, or strict diets. These trends, while well-intentioned, can weaken digestion, lower metabolism, and leave us feeling depleted because winter is a time for nourishment and restoration, not restriction and output.

In contrast, in the Southern Hemisphere, January is mid-summer, when energy is outward, temperatures are high, and digestion is naturally stronger. The body craves lighter, hydrating foods like fruits, salads, and cooling herbs. While this can be a more appropriate time for gentle detoxing or lighter eating, extreme restrictions in summer can still lead to imbalances, fatigue, and burnout, especially if done without considering the body's actual needs or hydration levels in the heat.

No matter where you are in the world, It is helpful to remember that spring-March/April in the North and September/October in the South are when the body is naturally ready to cleanse, reset, and shift toward lighter, fresh foods. This is when nature renews, and our digestion, energy, and clarity often follow suit. It is the ideal time to gently introduce new habits, healthier routines, and lighter meals without the stress or strain that can come from forcing those changes out of sync with the season.

By listening to the body and eating in alignment with the Earth's natural rhythm, we not only support digestion and energy but also create a more sustainable relationship with food and self-care. When we eat in season, we nourish more than our bodies-we restore balance in our entire system.

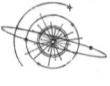# Mind: How Seasonal Energy Affects Mood and Mental Health

The changing seasons deeply influence the mind, especially during the colder, darker months. In the Northern Hemisphere, winter brings shorter days, limited sunlight, and colder temperatures, impacting the brain's natural chemistry. During this time, serotonin and dopamine, the feel-good neurotransmitters, drop. This can result in decreased mood, lower motivation, poor concentration, and increased fatigue.

January, in particular, can be an emotionally challenging time. It is the peak of winter and also the peak season for Seasonal Affective Disorder (SAD), a type of depression caused by lack of sunlight and disrupted circadian rhythms. Yet, despite this natural slowdown, modern culture continues to push for high productivity and dramatic resolutions. The result is a disconnect between the body's call for rest and society's demand for performance. This often leads to procrastination, guilt, burnout, and emotional exhaustion.

However, January lands mid-summer in the Southern Hemisphere- a season of long days, heat, light, and outward energy. While this time may feel more energising on the surface, it comes with mental and emotional challenges. The intense pace and stimulation of summer combined with holidays, social obligations, and heat stress can lead to overexertion, restlessness, emotional overload, or anxiety. The mind may feel scattered rather than focused, and some people feel pressure to perform or "make the most" of the season, even if they're internally craving calm or direction.

So, whether you are in the depths of winter (North) or the heights of summer (South), both extremes can create mental and emotional tension when not balanced with awareness and self-compassion. Pushing through major goals or life changes during these seasonal changes, especially without attuning to your own energy, leads to stress, disconnection, and inner resistance.

The key is to honour your mind's natural rhythm in harmony with the season. That may mean embracing rest and reflection in winter or slowing down and grounding yourself amid the high energy of summer. When we align our mental pace with nature's rhythm, we feel more balanced, resilient, and clear- no matter which side of the Earth we are on.

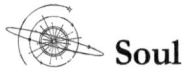 **Soul**

Nature moves in a sacred rhythm - a cycle of rest, renewal, action, and release. When we align ourselves with this rhythm, we find a deeper sense of ease, clarity, and connection. But when we push against it, especially in the name of productivity or self-improvement, we can become disconnected not just from nature but from ourselves.

Here is how the seasons guide our energy:

Winter
- It is a season of rest and reflection, a time for hibernation, deep thinking, and gentle slowing. It invites us to turn inward and replenish.

Spring
- A time of growth and renewal. Nature awakens, energy rises, and new beginnings feel natural. This is when our bodies and spirits align with action and fresh starts.

Summer
- It is a season of expansion and full expression. Creativity peaks, energy is vibrant, and we are in flow with productivity and outward momentum.

Autumn
- It is a time of harvest and preparation, where we gather wisdom, reflect on what we have created, and begin to slow down, making space for rest ahead.

When we force new beginnings in January - in the heart of winter - we skip the resting phase our bodies deeply crave. This disconnection from nature's timing can leave us exhausted, unmotivated, or resistant to change. The same thing happens in the Southern Hemisphere when we try to start fresh in September, during spring's fast-moving energy. In both cases, we are moving out of sync with the flow.

If you have ever felt low, foggy, or stuck during these times, know this: It is not your fault. Your body is wise. It is listening to the Earth's rhythm. The challenge is that modern society doesn't-it imposes artificial schedules and expectations that pull us away from the natural cycles, making life feel more draining and disorienting than it needs to be.

But here's the good news: when we begin to realign with the rhythm of nature, everything starts to shift. Goal-setting becomes gentler and more intuitive. Growth feels sustainable instead of forced. By syncing your intentions with the Earth's seasonal energies-governed by what many call Cosmic Flow-you begin to live with more harmony, purpose, and peace. You honour yourself. You honour the Earth. And you create space for a life that flows-not one that forces.

Just as nature follows a cyclical pattern of growth - planting, cultivating, harvesting, and resting - our lives can benefit from a similar rhythm of intention, action, reflection, and renewal. This perspective encourages seasonal awareness, deepening our spiritual and mental connection to the planet. Unlike the artificial constructs of the Gregorian calendar, which impose arbitrary deadlines and expectations, nature's cycles provide an intuitive and supportive framework for growth. Embracing this perspective leads to a more holistic way of living that recognises the interconnectedness of all things and promotes a sustainable, meaningful approach to personal development.

Manifestation, at its core, is about bringing our intentions and desires into reality through conscious thought, emotional alignment, action, and living intentionally - aligning ourselves with the rhythms of nature. By recognising that each season has its energy and purpose - whether it is the fresh beginnings of spring, the nurturing phase of summer, the completion of autumn, or the rest and reflection of winter - we can structure our actions and mindset to work in harmony with these natural cycles. This alignment helps us stay focused and grounded, deepening our connection to the earth and our growth journey.

When we live with this awareness, we empower ourselves to make conscious choices, honouring the flow of life rather than forcing outcomes. By trusting in the timing of the seasons, we create space for our desires to unfold naturally.

Embrace the seasons as your guide - plant your intentions, nourish them with effort, celebrate your harvests, and rest when needed. Trust that everything is unfolding in its perfect time, and know that you are always in sync with the cycles of the Cosmos.

Neuroscientific research also suggests that humans are biologically wired to respond positively to seasonal changes.

A study published in "Nature Communications" found that the brain's dopamine (reward) system is more active in the spring and summer months, leading to higher levels of motivation, optimism, and overall well-being.

This aligns with the practice of setting intentions in March, April, May, when the body's natural energy levels begin to rise, making it easier to take inspired action toward goals.

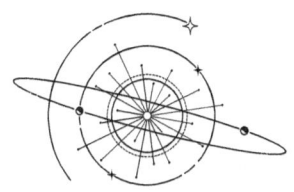

Training Your Brain

The brain you were born with is not the brain you die with! Not only are you programming it from the moment you were born, but you can also change and rewire it at any point in life - this is called neuroplasticity, the brain's remarkable ability to change, rewire, and adapt throughout your life.

Contrary to old beliefs that the brain stops developing after childhood, modern neuroscience has shown that our brains remain flexible and responsive to experience well into adulthood. Every thought, emotion and action you think activates neural pathways in the brain. When repeated often enough, these pathways become stronger - just like muscles being trained. Over time, this rewiring process can change how you think, feel, behave, and even how your body responds to stress.

This ability means healing, learning, and personal transformation are always possible. Whether you want to overcome anxiety, shift limiting beliefs, build confidence, or become more present, the brain can support that change - if given consistent input. This is the foundation for many modern therapeutic, coaching, and mindfulness practices. When we consciously engage with our thoughts and behaviours, we are not just creating change - we are rewiring our brains to sustain it.

So what we think - really matters!

We have 60,000 to 80,000 thoughts per day, with researchers estimating that about 80% to 90% of those are the same thoughts you had yesterday! And they will be 80-90% of the thoughts you have tomorrow unless you make a conscious effort to make a change.

These thoughts evoke approximately 400 distinct emotional experiences per day - positive or negative - some lasting only a few seconds, but some lasting hours, weeks, or even months. Many of these emotions release chemicals in the body, which can have a positive or negative effect. So, if you do not make a change, you can end up in a loop not only of thoughts but also of feelings and chemical releases in the body. So what you think is very important.

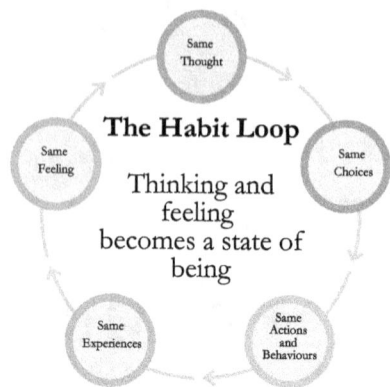

Example: Mindless Social Media Scrolling
Cue: You feel bored or stressed. And make the same choice
Routine: You grab your phone and open Instagram/TikTok.
Reward: You get a quick hit of entertainment or distraction, maybe a dopamine boost from likes or funny videos.

This kind of loop is super common - the reward satisfies the craving for stimulation or escape, so your brain keeps reinforcing it. But not all habit loops are negative.

Example: Confidence Habit Loop
Cue: You catch yourself doubting or second-guessing something
Routine: Pause → stand or sit tall → say out loud (or in your mind): "I trust myself. I do not need to be perfect to be powerful."
Reward: A boost of clarity, self-assurance, and grounded energy

Example: Daily Confidence Loop (5-Min Ritual)
Cue: After brushing your teeth in the morning
Routine: Look in the mirror
Say 3 affirmations:
"I trust myself." - "I can handle challenges." - "I belong in the rooms I enter."
Smile at yourself for 5 seconds
Reward: You start your day with self-anchoring energy and positive neural priming

Daily Practices to Rewire the Brain Using Neuroplasticity
Here are a few simple, science-backed practices that use neuroplasticity to help shift your mindset and emotional patterns over time:

 Gratitude Journaling (5 Minutes Daily)
Write down three things you are grateful for every day. The act of noticing what's good trains your brain to focus on the positive and builds new pathways associated with appreciation and joy.

Why it works: Repeated focus on gratitude rewires the brain for optimism and emotional resilience.

 Visualisation and Emotion (5–10 Minutes Daily)
Close your eyes and imagine a future version of yourself already living your desired life. Feel the emotions you would feel - confidence, peace, excitement, etc. Let those feelings fill your body.

Why it works: The brain doesn't distinguish well between real and vividly imagined experiences. This primes your neural pathways for success and builds emotional familiarity with your goals.

 Affirmations (2–3 Minutes Daily)
Repeat empowering statements that align with your goals (e.g., "I am grounded and confident," "I trust myself"). Say them slowly and with conviction, feeling the words in your body.

Why it works: Repeated statements, especially when felt emotionally, help replace old beliefs with new ones over time.

 Catch and Redirect (All Day Practice)
Notice negative self-talk or limiting thoughts when they arise. Pause, name the pattern ("That's the old belief"), and choose a more supportive thought.

Why it works: Each time you interrupt an old thought loop and choose a new one, you weaken the old pathway and strengthen the new one.

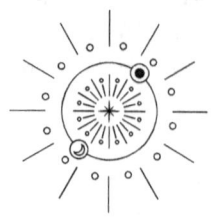

Neuroplasticity reminds us that we are not fixed. With small, intentional actions, you can literally rewire your brain to support who you are becoming. Consistency matters more than intensity - because every repetition is a vote for the future you.

Teanna

From the moment you were born, you have been programming your brain through every experience you have had. Even if you cannot remember the actual event, the emotional responses are stored for future use, regardless of whether the experience was real or not. The sad thing is that research has shown that we embellish memory and that only 50% of what we remember from the past is true - so many people can be stuck in a negative habit loop based on memories that have not actually happened!

The brain also cannot always distinguish between real and imagined, nor can it, at first, easily tell the difference between what is safe and what is a threat. Take the fear of spiders - a common phobia in the UK. Realistically, there are no deadly spiders in the UK, and spider bites are extremely rare. Yet many people are terrified of them. Why? This is likely because, at some point, they saw a parent or peer react fearfully to a spider. That reaction created an emotional imprint, and they have adopted the same fear - even though a spider has never harmed them. This is a classic case of learned behaviour and an irrational fear that has now been stored in the brain. Furthermore, the chemical Adrenaline (fight-or-flight) is released whenever they see a spider and every time this happens, it reinforces the experience in the brain repeatedly - until the pattern is intentionally broken.

Many of our irrational imprints are formed before the age of six, as during that time, the brain operates primarily in theta waves - a deeply receptive state ideal for unconscious learning and programming. (see page 59 re brainwaves) This is when we form core beliefs about ourselves and the world - like "I am not good enough" or "I am only loved when I perform". These beliefs can stick into adulthood as 'irrational imprints' or 'emotional triggers', even if we are unaware of them. Around the age of seven, the brain shifts out of the dominant theta wave state and starts operating more in alpha and beta brainwaves. This transition marks a move from subconscious absorption to more conscious thinking, logic, and reasoning.

We begin to develop a stronger sense of self-awareness, critical thinking, and the ability to analyse information rather than absorb it. This is also when the conscious mind becomes more active, and learning becomes more intentional rather than purely experiential.

In short, the brain starts functioning more like an adult's - still growing, but now with more conscious control and mental structure. As the brain develops into adulthood, it moves into a more stable pattern of beta wave dominance, which supports focused attention, problem-solving, decision-making, and goal-oriented thinking.

During adolescence, the prefrontal cortex - the part responsible for reasoning, impulse control, and planning - continues to mature. This process is not fully complete until the mid-20s, which is why teens often act on emotion or impulse.

Over time, repeated thoughts, emotional responses, and behaviours become deeply wired into the brain, forming automatic patterns the mind relies on for efficiency. By age 35, most people live primarily from their subconscious programming, meaning their thoughts, behaviours, emotional reactions, and habits have become deeply automatic. As a result, around 90–95% of daily actions and reactions occur on autopilot, often without conscious thought. People tend to wake up, think the same thoughts, feel the same emotions, and repeat the same routines-essentially reliving their past each day.

While the brain is still capable of change, transformation requires intentional effort by this age. Rewiring these ingrained patterns involves conscious awareness, new habits, and consistent practice, but the good news is that lasting change is entirely possible with effort. We can rewire habits, change beliefs, and reshape our emotional responses at any age. This is essentially what Manifestation is - making changes to your life by reprogramming your brain.

The first step to change is deciding to do so and creating meaningful intentions. The second step is evoking emotions related to those intentions. When you do this, you are programming the Reticular Activating System (RAS) to start noticing related opportunities, synchronises, co-incidences, and patterns.

The RAS is a network of neurons in the brain stem. The brain's filter decides what gets your attention and what fades into the background, and you can program it to work for you. For example, if you focus on abundance, you will see more opportunities for success. If you focus on limitations, the RAS will highlight obstacles instead.

For example, whenever you have bought a new car, You will have gone through a process of looking for one logical process, probably weighing up the pros and cons.

But at some point, you made a decision and attached emotion to it. You may even compromise on one of your desired feature lists. But at this point that you attached emotion, your RAS understood that these thoughts you were having were important - and guess what - you started to see lots of the make and model of the car you had chosen on the road around you!

This is exactly how the emotional part of manifesting works. Those cars have always been there - the natural flow of energy puts them there every day; you just do not see them. But once you had set a meaningful intention to buy a new car AND attached emotion to it, the RAS started to point them out to you.

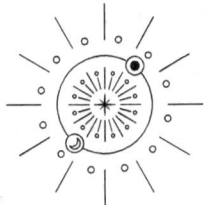

"In its simplest form, the brain is just a record of the past"

Teanna

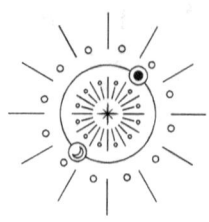

*"Manifestation is not just about wishful thinking.
It is deeply connected to how the brain processes thoughts, beliefs, and emotions to shape reality.*

The brain plays a key role in visualisation, focus, belief systems, and action-taking, all of which influence manifestation."

Teanna

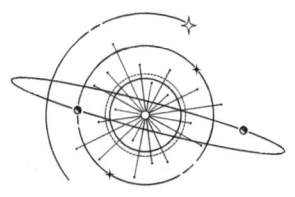

Meditation and the Brain

Meditation is nothing new; it has existed for thousands of years in recorded history. Indian artefacts have proven a form of meditation called "Tantra," dating back over 5,000 years. Researchers even suggest that primitive hunter-gatherers may have been the ones to discover meditation and its many different states of consciousness while gazing into the flames of their fires.

Of course, the Buddha is known as one of the most prominent meditation icons and has existed since 500 B.C. However, its popularity in the West started in the mid-20th century when researchers in the 1960s and 1970s started to learn about its medical benefits.

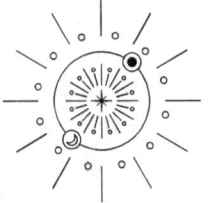

"In its simplest form meditation is a practice that helps people achieve balance - mentally, physically and emotionally"

Teanna

We all know relaxation is beneficial to health, yet we all know that you cannot just switch a switch to relax, but we can meditate - and it is free :) You can practice it at home or join a local meditation group. In time, you can even do it on the train as you commute - you will discover the benefits no matter how you incorporate meditation into your life.

Meditation helps lower your heart rate and blood pressure by slowing your breathing. This reduces the amount of oxygen needed for the body. The thought process allows the mind and muscles to relax gently.

As the saying goes, "If you are too busy for 10 minutes daily, you should meditate for 20 minutes". But honestly, even 2 minutes will bring benefits - if you start with a tiny habit and consistently achieve it, it will grow.

There are different ways to meditate

Meditation comes in many forms, each catering to different needs, mindsets, and spiritual traditions. Mindfulness meditation, rooted in Buddhism, focuses on staying present and observing thoughts without judgment. Mantra meditation, commonly practised in Hinduism, involves repeating sacred sounds like "Om" or "So Hum" to deepen concentration and align with higher consciousness. Guided meditation uses visualisation and spoken guidance to relax the mind and manifest desired outcomes. Transcendental meditation (TM) involves silently repeating a personal mantra to reach a deep, restful awareness. Movement-based meditations like yoga, tai chi, and walking meditation integrate breath and physical movement to create a meditative flow state. Loving-kindness meditation (Metta) focuses on cultivating compassion and sending positive energy to oneself and others. Trataka (candle-gazing meditation) improves focus by staring at a flame, whilst breath work meditations like Pranayama regulate emotions through controlled breathing techniques. Each method provides unique benefits, allowing individuals to choose the practice that resonates most with their journey toward inner peace and self-awareness.

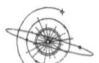

Which is the best?

All meditation is good, but some people prefer a particular method.

- **Mindfulness Meditation** involves sitting quietly and noticing your thoughts without judgment. It is the most popular and versatile form of meditation and is great for beginners. It is perfect for stress relief, anxiety, clarity, and emotional balance.

- **Guided Meditation** is the easiest to start with. It is where you listen to a recorded voice or a live teacher who leads you through visualisation, relaxation, or intention-setting. This is great for beginners, overthinkers, or those who need structure.

- **Loving-Kindness (Metta) Meditation** involves sending kindness to yourself and others through phrases like "May I be happy, may you be well." This practice is good for healing, compassion, forgiveness, and self-love and is surprisingly powerful, especially if you are feeling down or disconnected.

- **Focused Attention Meditation** involves focusing on one thing - a mantra, the breath, a candle flame, etc. It is best for training concentration and calming a restless mind. It is good if you like structure or get easily distracted.

- **Transcendental Meditation (TM)** involves silently repeating a specific mantra for 20 minutes twice a day. It is best for deep rest, reducing anxiety, and unlocking creativity. This method requires the mantra to be given to you by a TM facilitator, you usually pays for it. However, you can also find these online.

- **Walking or Movement Meditation** is a gentle, mindful movement, like tai chi or yoga. It is best for people who find sitting still difficult and is excellent for grounding and connecting to your body.

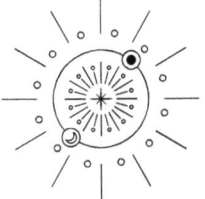

*" In stillness,
I listen.
In presence,
I bloom."*

Teanna

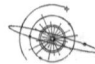 ## What happens in your brain when you meditate?

When we meditate, our brain waves, some lobes and brain organs change. These can be seen using big hospital MRIs and small head scanners like the Muse headband. Even if you have never tried meditation before and think you have failed, after a single 20-minute meditation session, your brain will have slowed down, and the MRI scan will show this.

We have five major brain waves, and the calmer we become, the lower our frequency gets with each wave, which is measured in hertz (Hz). Brain waves are electrical impulses in the brain that occur due to the communication between neurons. They are patterns of neural oscillations that correspond to different mental states, such as focus, relaxation, sleep, and heightened alertness, and all operate at different Hz.

1 Delta Wave (0.5 to 4 Hz)
- These are low, high-amplitude waves associated with restorative sleep and healing. They are most prevalent during deep, dreamless sleep and unconscious states.

2 Theta Wave (4 to 8 Hz)
- This one is associated with vivid imagery, intuition, and daydreaming. It is active during light sleep, deep meditation, and moments of creativity.

3 Alpha Wave (8 to 12 Hz)
- This indicates a relaxed awareness, often linked to a meditative state. It is active during quiet, resting states, such as when you close your eyes and relax.

4 Beta Wave (12 to 30 Hz)
- This is dominant during conscious activities like problem-solving, decision-making, and social interaction.

5 Gamma Wave (30 to 100 Hz)
- This one is associated with high-level cognitive functioning, learning, and peak focus and is most active during complex problem-solving, moments of insight, and deep learning.

In addition to the five widely recognised brain waves, lesser-known or more recently proposed brain waves may also play a role in higher consciousness, sensory integration, and motor functions.

These additional waves include Lambda Waves (100-200 Hz), which have been linked to heightened sensory perception, rapid cognitive processing, and deep states of meditation; Epsilon Waves (<0.5 Hz), which are theorised to occur in the deepest states of meditation and transcendental consciousness, possibly serving as the extreme low-frequency counterpart to Gamma waves; and Hyper-Gamma Waves (100-200 Hz) are believed to be associated with advanced intuition, problem-solving, and spiritual experiences. Another notable brain wave pattern is the Mu Wave (8-13 Hz), which is connected to motor control, mirror neuron activity, and social learning and often becomes suppressed when an individual engages in movement or action.

While the five major brain waves are well-documented in neuroscience, these additional waves remain an area of ongoing research, particularly in meditation, consciousness studies, and neuroplasticity. Their roles in perception, cognition, and self-awareness are still being explored.

Human Brain Anatomy

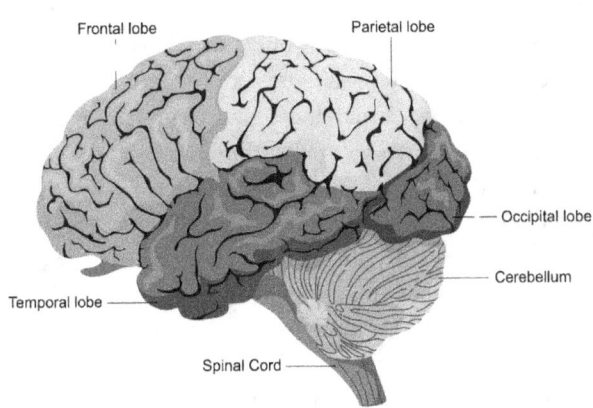

Meditation also changes the activity in our lobes, especially the 'Prefrontal Cortex'. This is the most highly evolved part of the brain, responsible for reasoning, planning, emotions, and self-conscious awareness. During meditation, the frontal cortex switches off.

Activity in the 'Parietal' lobe slows down. This part of the brain processes sensory information about the surrounding world, orienting you in time and space.

Meditation also reduces the flow of incoming information in the 'Thalamus' to a trickle. The Thalamus is not a lobe but an organ inside the brain that is the gatekeeper of the senses. This organ focuses your attention by funnelling some sensory data more profoundly into the brain and stopping other signals.

Meditating also dials back the arousal signal via the 'Reticulated Formation'; as the brain's sentry, this structure receives incoming stimuli and puts the brain on alert, ready to respond.

Interestingly, when you meditate daily, your brain continues in this state even when you are awake and going about your daily business - call it inner peace if you wish. Getting to this state takes time, but it is a beautiful place to be.

Also, the more we meditate, the less anxiety we have because we loosen the connections of particular neural pathways in the 'Medial Prefrontal Cortex' (sometimes called the Me Centre). This part of the brain processes information relating to ourselves and our experiences, and it gets tighter over time.

For example, when we experience a scary or upsetting sensation, it triggers a strong reaction in our 'Me Centre', making us feel scared and under attack. When we meditate, we weaken this neural connection. This means that we do not react as strongly to sensations that might have once lit up our ' Me Centre'. As we weaken this connection, we simultaneously strengthen the connection between what is known as our 'Assessment Centre' (the part of our brain known for reasoning) and our bodily sensation and fear centres. So, when we experience scary or upsetting sensations again, we can more easily look at them rationally. For example, when you experience pain, rather than becoming anxious and assuming it means something is wrong with you, you can watch the pain rise and fall without becoming ensnared in a story about what it might mean.

Research on meditation has shown that those who practice meditation regularly have higher empathy and compassion. One experiment showed the participants images of other people who were either good, bad, or neutral in what they called "compassion meditation." The participants could focus their attention and "reduce their emotional reactions to these images, even when they were not in a meditative state." They also experienced more compassion for others when shown disturbing images.

Part of this comes from activity in the 'Amygdala' - the part of the brain that processes emotional stimuli. During meditation, this part of the brain usually shows decreased activity, but in this experiment, it was exceptionally responsive when participants were shown images of people.

Another study in 2008 found that people who meditated regularly had more substantial activation levels in their 'Temporal Parietal Junctures' (a part of the brain tied to empathy) when they heard the sounds of people suffering than those who did not.

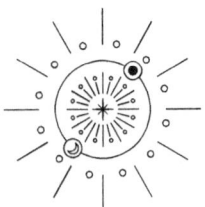

"Meditation not only gave me my life back! It gave me my soul purpose"

Teanna

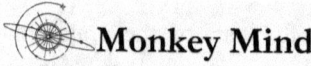 Monkey Mind

Intrusive thoughts in meditation are natural, unwanted, involuntary thoughts that disrupt focus and can be distracting, repetitive, or even distressing. They often take the form of random memories, worries, negative self-talk, or irrational fears. These thoughts arise because the mind naturally seeks stimulation, and unconscious thoughts surface when meditation slows mental activity. Stress and anxiety can also make them more frequent. Most meditation facilitators would advise that the best way to handle intrusive thoughts is to 'acknowledge' them without resistance, label them as 'thinking' or 'worrying', and gently return to your focus, whether it is the breath, a mantra, or bodily sensations. I prefer a technique of 'giving them to your Monkey'- A hypothetical monkey inside your head or on your shoulder - to which you give the thought. This metaphor is your subconscious brain, which will hold the thought.

The key is not to judge yourself but to practice self-compassion. Over time, these thoughts lose their power, and meditation becomes a greater clarity and calm space.

'Giving them to your Monkey' also links to the idea of a 'Monkey mind', a term from Buddhist teachings that describes a restless, unsettled, and easily distracted state of mind in which thoughts jump around like a monkey swinging from tree to tree.

"Meditation is a practice... the more you practice the easier it will become"

Teanna

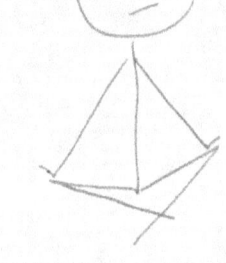

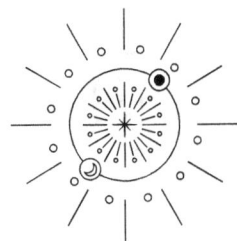

"If you want to find the secrets of the universe, think in terms of energy, frequency, and vibration"

Nikola Tesla

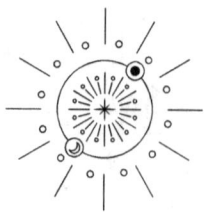

*"Aligning manifestation
to natural
energy cycles,
stops manifestation
being
a process or an exercise -
it becomes
a way of life."*

Teanna

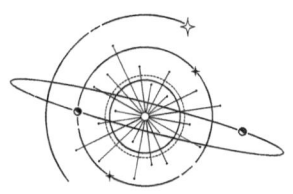

Brain and Heart Coherence

For centuries, the heart has been seen as the seat of emotion, intuition, and memory. While this idea has often been symbolic or poetic, modern science is now exploring whether there might be more truth than we once believed.

Research has confirmed that the heart is far more intelligent than a simple pump. It contains around 40,000 neurons, forming what scientists call the intrinsic cardiac nervous system - essentially a "little brain in the heart." This system can process information, learn, and even remember in fundamental ways, all while communicating constantly with the brain via the vagus nerve.

One of the most intriguing pieces of evidence comes from heart transplant recipients. There are several documented cases where individuals report changes in personality, habits, or emotional responses after receiving a new heart. Some begin craving foods their donors loved or develop talents or fears they never had before. Though these stories are anecdotal and not yet scientifically proven, they raise the possibility of cellular memory - the idea that information can be stored in the cells of organs, not just the brain.

In addition, studies from the HeartMath Institute show that the heart's rhythm patterns can affect brain function, especially in areas related to emotional processing and memory. When in a state of heart coherence - a smooth, harmonious rhythm often linked with positive emotions - the heart actually helps regulate our mental and emotional states.

While mainstream science has not confirmed that the heart stores memory in the same way the brain does, the evidence is growing that the heart plays a critical role in how we process, store, and even embody emotional experiences. The conversation is shifting - from the heart as metaphor to the heart as a true source of intelligence.

In addition, the connection between the heart and brain is deeply tied to emotional processing. Research has shown that the rhythms of the heart - especially when we are experiencing emotions like gratitude, love, or appreciation - can affect brain functions related to memory and decision-making. While this does not mean the heart stores memories like the brain, it does suggest the heart plays a role in how we process and recall emotional experiences.

When it comes to manifesting, the harmony between your brain and heart plays a deeply powerful role. At its core, manifestation is about aligning your thoughts and emotions with what you want to create or attract in your life. When your brain - which governs your thoughts and intentions - and your heart - the center of your emotions and feelings - are in

The Girl Who Dreamed of Her Donor's Killer

Eight-year-old Danielle was just beginning to recover from a life-threatening heart condition when she received a donor heart from another young girl. The surgery went smoothly, and doctors were thrilled with her physical progress. But soon after the transplant, something unexpected happened.

Danielle began having vivid, recurring nightmares. In the dreams, she saw a man chasing a girl through the woods, grabbing her, and hurting her. She described the attacker in chilling detail: his face, clothing, the way he spoke, even the exact location where the attack happened. The dreams became so intense that her parents brought her to a psychiatrist, concerned about her mental health.

What happened next stunned everyone.

At the psychiatrist's suggestion, the parents and medical team contacted the police - and they discovered that Danielle's donor had been murdered. Even more shocking: the description Danielle gave matched the actual crime scene, including details that had never been made public. Acting on her testimony, the police were able to identify and eventually convict the man who had taken the donor's life.

sync, you enter a state of alignment that supports the manifestation process.
As shared before, manifesting is not just about thinking positively. It requires both clear intention and an elevated emotional state.

The brain forms the mental image - the vision of what you want - while the heart provides the emotional fuel that energises that vision. When you reach a state of coherence, your heart and brain communicate clearly, allowing you to actually feel the emotion of already having what you desire. That feeling begins to shape your external reality.

The heart is a key player here - it produces the most powerful electromagnetic field in the body, even stronger than the brain's. When you are in heart coherence, that field becomes more stable, ordered, and focused. In manifestation terms, you send a clear, intentional, energetic signal into the cosmos. Therefore, that emotional frequency helps draw in experiences that match your internal state.

On the flip side, if you are trying to manifest something - like love, success, or peace - but feeling anxious, doubtful, or fearful, your heart and brain are out of sync. That disconnect between your heart and brain creates resistance, and it can block the very things you're trying to call in. Coherence shifts you into a more open, receptive state where your thoughts and feelings align, and your energy matches the reality you want to create.

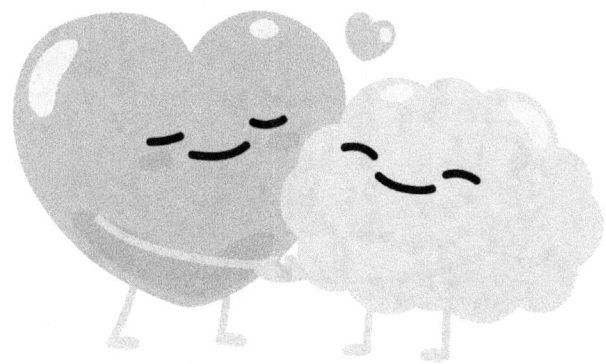

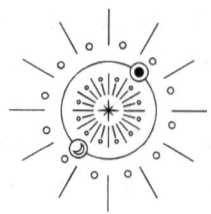

"The first step is simple but profound: Let go of January and embrace Spring as your true New Year"

Teanna

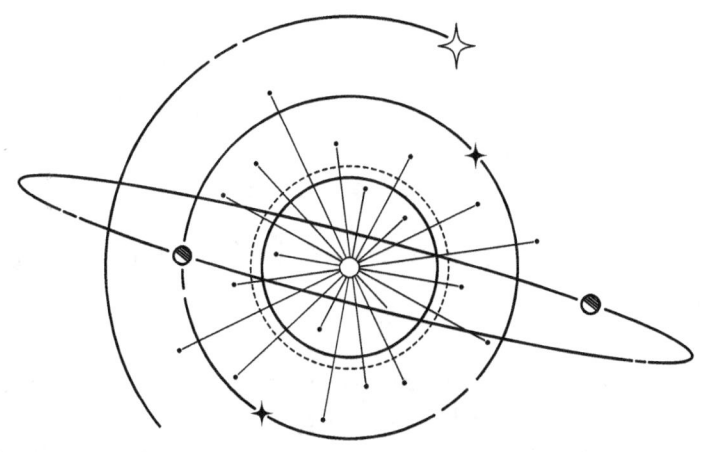

Manifesting with Cosmic Flow

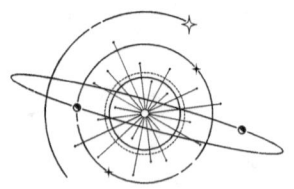

How Long Does it Take to Manifest?

The time it takes for a manifestation to materialise varies from person to person and depends on several factors, including clarity of intention, emotional alignment, belief system, resistance levels, and divine timing. There is no fixed timeline, but understanding these key influences can help you trust the process and stay aligned with the flow. Some manifestations happen instantly, while others require patience and personal growth before they appear. When this becomes a way of life, it flows with ease.

One of the most significant factors affecting manifestation speed is clarity of intention. The Cosmos responds more quickly when you are specific and clear about what you want. Vague desires create unclear energy, leading to delays. Another crucial element is emotional alignment - the more you feel gratitude, joy, and confidence, as if your manifestation is already here, the faster it can arrive. However, if you are consumed by doubt, fear, or a sense of lack, these emotions create resistance, slowing the process.

Your belief system also plays a significant role. If you genuinely believe you deserve what you manifest and that it is possible, it will come more quickly. On the other hand, if you have limiting beliefs such as "I am not worthy of success" or "Good things never happen to me," these thoughts create barriers that take time to dissolve. Resistance and attachment can further delay manifestations - constantly worrying about "When will it happen?" or feeling desperate can block the natural flow of energy. Surrendering and trusting the flow allows things to unfold effortlessly.

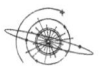
Estimated Time-Frames for Manifestation

- **Instant** (Minutes to Days): Small manifestations, such as seeing angel numbers, finding a parking spot, or receiving a quick sign from the Cosmos, often happen fast because of little resistance.

- **Short-Term** (Days to Weeks): When you fully align, deeply believe in your manifestation, and take inspired action, results can appear quickly.

- **Medium-Term** (Weeks to Months): Bigger manifestations, like career changes, attracting a soulmate, or financial growth, often require inner shifts, preparation, and external alignment before they materialise.

- **Long-Term** (Months to Years): Life-changing manifestations, such as a dream home, massive career success, or profound spiritual transformation, can take longer as they involve major energetic shifts, lessons, and divine timing.

 How to Speed Up the Process:
- Be clear and specific - Set a firm, precise intention
- Embody the emotions now - Feel as if it has already happened
- Release resistance - Let go of attachment and trust the process
- Follow inspired action - Act when you feel nudged, without force
- Stay patient and in flow - Avoid desperation and trust in divine timing

The following chapters will discuss each of these in-depth, but remember, manifestation is not about forcing things to happen but about aligning yourself with what is already meant for you. When you stop worrying about how long it will take and focus on becoming someone who already has it, things unfold naturally and often faster than expected.

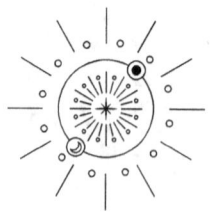

"Manifestation does not happen on your schedule - it happens when your energy aligns with your desire. Trust the timing."

Teanna

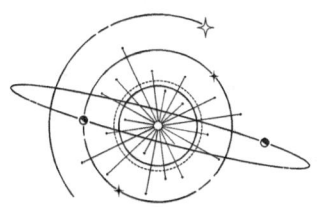

6 steps to Manifesting with Cosmic Flow

 Align yourself with the natural flow of the seasonal energies

 Review and Reflect
Where are you now, and where are you going? You should ask this at every change of season to make sure you are still on the right path with the new knowledge you have gained. For deeper internal work, use the Cosmic energy of winter.

Set Your Intentions
These should be clear and concise. Small intentions can be set at any time, but for big life-changing intentions, use the Cosmic energy of spring.

 Emotional Alignment
This is the most important step. You have to truly feel the emotions in order to train your brain and heart to see the opportunities the Cosmos will put in your path. This should be done <u>all</u> the time - power boosts will come with each full moon. For deep emotional work use the Cosmic energy boost of spring, summer and autumn.

 Trust and Flow
Surrender, allowing the Cosmos to unfold events perfectly and show you the opportunities and synchronicity around you.

 Inspired Action
Act on these opportunities, synchronicities, co-incidents and intuitive nudges but without force. These could appear at any time

The 'Cosmic Flow Method' blends intentional manifestation through neuroscience with trust, surrender, and intuitive alignment, all in flow with the natural energy cycles - the natural flow of Cosmic Energy. It helps you manifest by aligning your energy with that of the Cosmos via setting clear, meaningful intentions, evoking emotions, training your brain away from limiting beliefs and allowing the flow to guide the process to opportunities and synchronicities. All of this aligns with the natural energy given to us via the natural cycles of the Cosmos, the sun, the moon, and the seasonal cycles.

There are a few components I wish to share with you: the actual stages of manifestation and the methods to shift your energy, reprogram your subconscious, and align with new possibilities. Also, I learned how to use the cosmic energy available in each season. I will talk you through all of these in the following chapters, and I have also put together four seasonal-based workbooks to hold your hand for a whole year per season, with weekly exercises - nothing overbearing or overwhelming, just a nice flow to awaken your awareness to the energy flow and the principles of manifesting. With a balanced approach to your personal energy levels and those of the Cosmos.

Understanding the principal steps of manifestation and the methods to shift your energy, reprogram your subconscious, and align with new possibilities is fundamental. First, I would like to introduce you to the energy cycles of the seasons.

Living by the principles of manifestation means constantly setting clear intentions, embodying emotions including gratitude and abundance, surrendering control, and trusting divine timing. Rather than reacting to life with frustration, fear, or doubt, you begin to see every experience - positive or challenging - as part of your path. You trust everything is unfolding exactly as it should, even if you cannot see the bigger picture. Over time, this trust strengthens, and manifestation becomes second nature rather than something you must consciously practice.

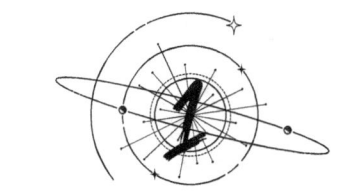

Align with Cosmic Energy

The key to making manifestation a way of life is aligning to the natural energy of the Cosmos, the Earth and nature and aligning your thoughts, emotions, and actions with the reality you want to experience. It means embodying the person you aspire to be, not waiting for external circumstances to change. It is about choosing abundance over lack, love over fear, and faith over doubt in every situation. The more you practice this, the easier it becomes, and soon, you will notice that the things you once struggled to manifest come to you effortlessly.

By adopting manifestation as a lifestyle, you move in harmony with the seasons of life, embracing cycles of growth, refinement, and transformation. You understand that ...

...everything happens in divine timing and that your role is not to control but to trust, flow and take inspired action when the moment is right.

Teanna

Cosmic energy is given to us in natural seasons, each with a unique energy and purpose - spring for sowing seeds, summer for cultivating growth, autumn for gratitude and refining, and winter for inner transformation.

Following this cycle allows our desires to unfold in perfect divine timing with ease, flow and peace in your soul.

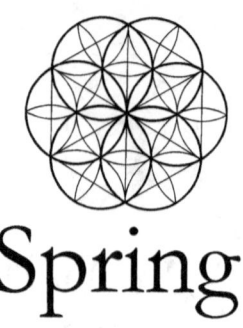

Spring

Spring is the season of 'Awakening' - a time when the natural world bursts into life after the stillness of winter. Flowers bloom, seeds sprout, and animals emerge from hibernation. The earth vibrates with energy, fertility, and potential. This season carries a unique vitality that invites renewal and growth, symbolising fresh beginnings. Just as the soil prepares to nurture new life, we can embrace this opportunity for transformation.

The power of spring for manifestation is backed by neuroscience. When we set intentions during a season characterised by growth and renewal, our brains are more receptive to creating new neural pathways. This is partly due to a natural surge in dopamine, the 'feel-good' neurotransmitter, which plays a crucial role in motivation and goal achievement. This neurotransmitter enhances focus and drive, making it easier to pursue our goals; even with small, achievable tasks, like organising a room or starting a new habit, we stimulate dopamine release, reinforcing our momentum and enthusiasm.

Spring also boosts serotonin levels, the neurotransmitter linked to mood regulation and emotional well-being. The increased exposure to sunlight and longer daylight hours naturally elevates serotonin, improving our mood, energy levels, and motivation. This seasonal uplift aligns our minds and bodies for growth, making it the perfect time to plant the seeds of our dreams.

Spring is more than just a season; it is a powerful reminder of the cycles of life, renewal, and infinite possibilities. By consciously aligning with this energy, we can manifest our dreams with greater ease and joy. Just as nature awakens, our aspirations can blossom and thrive.

Spring Workbook

During this season, the emphasis should be on learning to find your true intentions, set them, and refine them. It should also be an introduction to the other detailed practices of visualisation, affirmations, self-love, gratitude, and meditation, all included in the Spring workbook.

In Spring, you should take some time to reflect on your life purpose by doing the 'Ikigiai' (page 87) and then discover where you are in life right now via the 'Life Balance Wheel' (page 94). This is important so you know where you are now, where you want to go, and, thus, which direction to go.

Then, move to setting your intentions and creating an action plan for the basic steps you feel you need to take. This is only the first step or the first few at most - nothing like a complete path - as that is the whole point of manifestation; at some point, you must surrender, trust, and flow.

On page 104, visualisation techniques are explained, affirmations are covered on page 114 and gratitude on page 122.

Spring begins in March with the Spring Equinox and continues through April and May. This means that starting your manifestations on any day during these months will still align with the uplifting, growth-filled energy of the season. It is not about a single day - the entire season carries the momentum of renewal and new beginnings.

We also have three full moons, energy boosts, for which I have created a complete ritual; in April, we have the 'Pink Full Moon' named after early spring flowers like phlox, indicating renewal, blossoming, and the vibrancy of life. In May, the 'Flower Full Moon ' represents the abundant blooming of flowers, symbolising growth, beauty, and the flourishing of life. In June, there will be the 'Strawberry Full Moon', which marks the time to harvest ripening strawberries, symbolising abundance, fruition, and the sweetness of life. All of these have practical practices in the Spring workbook and online meditations.

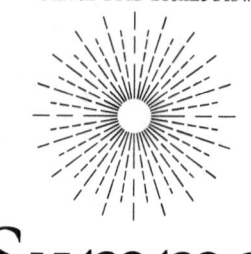

Summer

Summer is a season of vitality, abundance, and momentum when the natural world is fully blooming. The sun shines brightly, energy is at its peak, and growth is at its most visible. Flowers open, fruits ripen, and animals move with purpose, taking full advantage of the season's warmth and abundance. Just as nature thrives, in this phase of expansion, we, too, are called to step into bold action, confidence, and inspired creation.

The power of summer in manifestation lies in its active, high-energy frequency. This is the time to embody the reality of your manifestations entirely - not just dreaming or planning but living as if they are already yours. The seeds were planted in spring, and now, with summer's intensity, it is time to nurture, protect, and actively cultivate what we have set in motion. The Cosmos responds to action, and the summer's energy supports us in taking courageous steps forward in career, relationships, and personal growth.

Neurologically, summer is a season of dopamine-driven momentum. The long, sunlit days naturally boost serotonin and endorphin levels, enhancing our mood, focus, and energy. This makes it the perfect time for bold, inspired action - launching new projects, deepening connections, expanding opportunities, and embracing challenges with confidence.

Manifestation is not just about the destination but about experiencing the journey with excitement and gratitude. By soaking in the joy of the present moment, we amplify our energetic frequency, making us even more magnetic to our desires. So, while summer is an active season, it is also a time of joy, celebration, and presence. Just as nature does not rush but enjoys the fullness of each moment, we are reminded to savour the process.

Summer is more than just a season - it is an invitation to live boldly, act with confidence, and trust in the abundance of the Cosmos. By aligning with its energy we embrace the power of momentum, expansion, and fearless creation. As the sun fuels life, this season encourages us to shine, thrive, and take inspired steps toward our desired future.

 ## Summer Workbook

Summer is the season of growth, confidence, and action. It is the time to deepen our understanding of our true intentions - refining them, committing to them, and integrating them into our daily lives. While spring is about discovering our path, summer is about walking it with clarity and purpose.

If you worked through the 'Spring workbook - Sow Seeds of Success,' you have already explored the basic concepts of intention setting, visualisations, gratitude, aligned actions, and reflection. During the summer, these should become second nature, but I will still hold your hand through the process of action, reflection, and celebration.

During early summer, you should revisit the Ikigai exercise (page 87) to see if anything has changed. Have you learnt new skills? Have you gained any clarity? Found another hobby? Then, check in with your Life Balance Wheel (page 94) to reassess your current position in life. Just as nature is in full bloom, your goals should flourish with newfound clarity. Ask yourself: What intentions have taken root, and what adjustments must be made?

Once you have refined your intentions, develop an action plan with small, meaningful steps. Remember that manifestation is not about rigid control but setting your course and allowing space for flow, trust, and divine timing. Please take action. If the wish is insufficient, watch for the synchronicities and follow them. Visualisation techniques strengthen your ability to see, feel, and believe in your desired reality. Learn the 'Pomodoro Technique' (page 235), understand your 'Inner Critic vs. inner Coach' (page 238), and take bold steps on your action plan.

We start Summer with the 'Summer Solstice' in June, and we have three full moons, for which I have created a complete ritual. In July, we have the 'Buck Moon', with the energy of 'Strength and Confidence'. This moon coincides with the period when male deer grow new antlers, representing growth, strength, and renewal. Then, in August, we have the 'Sturgeon Moon', named by Native American tribes for the abundant sturgeon fish during this time. With the energy of 'Prosperity and Manifestation,' this moon symbolises the provision of resources. Then, finally, in October, there will be the 'Harvest Moon' with the energy of 'Reaping Rewards,' symbolising preparation for the coming winter. All of these have practical practices and online meditations.

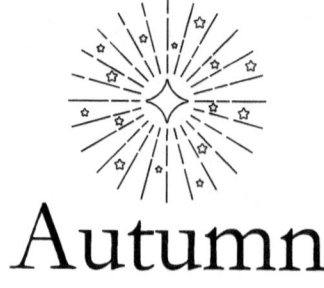

Autumn

Autumn is a season of harvest and transformation when the natural world shifts from the fullness of summer to a period of reflection and release. Leaves change colour and fall, symbolising the beauty of letting go. Crops are gathered, marking the rewards of past efforts, while the air carries a crisp reminder that a new cycle is approaching. Just as nature sheds what is no longer needed, we, too, are invited to reassess, refine, and realign our intentions and manifestations.

The power of autumn in manifestation lies in its energy of refinement. This is a time to take stock of your progress, acknowledge what is working, and release what is holding you back. Just as trees let go of their leaves to conserve energy for winter, we must let go of doubts, outdated beliefs, and distractions that no longer serve. This process is not about loss but about creating space for new possibilities. The more we release, the more we allow fresh energy and opportunities to flow into our lives.

Autumn is a time of increased mindfulness and reflection from a neurological perspective. As daylight hours shorten, our brain naturally becomes more introspective. The change in seasons encourages us to slow down, evaluate our choices, and make intentional adjustments. This is the perfect time to refine your goals, adjust your vision, and realign with what truly matters. This season, journaling, meditation, and gratitude practices become powerful tools, helping you integrate lessons from the past cycle and prepare for what is next.

Autumn also teaches us the balance between action and surrender. While it is a season of harvesting past efforts, it also reminds us that some things take longer to ripen. Not every seed planted in spring is ready for harvest, which is okay. The key is to trust the process - to appreciate the fruits of our labour while allowing what still needs time to evolve naturally.

More than just a season of transition, autumn is a sacred space for reflection, refinement and preparation. By consciously aligning with its energy, we learn to release what no longer serves us, honour the lessons of the past and set the stage for future manifestations. Just as nature gracefully transitions, we can embrace change with trust and wisdom, knowing that every shift guides us closer to our highest potential.

 ## Autumn Workbook

With the cooling air and slowing rhythm of nature, deepen your manifestation practice by embracing surrender, patience, and gratitude. Reflection and celebration are as critical as action, so acknowledge how far you have come and honour the lessons you have learned. Celebrate any wins, no matter how small, and then reflect, refine, and release.

As the trees shed their leaves, this is a time to let go of what no longer serves you, clearing space for new growth. If you worked through the Spring and Summer Workbooks, you have already explored intention setting, visualisation, affirmations, gratitude, and aligned action. Now, it is time to assess, adjust, and realign. So, revisit the Ikigai exercise (page 87) and Life Balance Wheel (page 94) during early Autumn. Has your path shifted? Have new experiences or realisations changed your vision? If so, now is the time for you to adjust your intentions.

Then, as the nights grow longer, practice self-inquiry and journaling to strengthen your inner wisdom. Work with release rituals, shadow work (on page 228), and more profound meditation to clear limiting beliefs and emotional blockages. Manifestation is not just about calling in what you desire but also about making space for it, changing these built-in belief systems, and creating new neural pathways.

We start Autumn with the Equinox in September and have three full moons this season. In October, the 'Hunter's Moon' signifies the time to hunt and prepare for winter, symbolising readiness, survival, and life cycle. With the energy of 'Focus and Determination'. Then, in November, we have the 'Beaver Moon', which indicates the time beavers build their dams, symbolising industriousness, preparation, and the onset of colder seasons. This moon has the energy of 'Preparation and Stability'. Then, in December, we have the 'Cold Moon' with the energy of 'Stillness and Reflection', which reflects December's long, cold nights. All of these have practical exercises and online meditations.

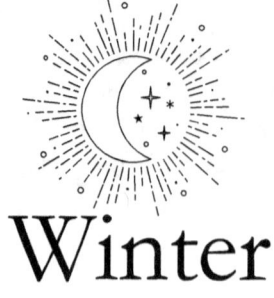

Winter

Winter is a season of stillness and introspection when the natural world slows down, conserving energy for the renewal that will follow. Trees shed their leaves, the earth rests beneath a blanket of frost, and animals retreat into hibernation. This season carries a unique energy of reflection, inner transformation, and deep alignment. Just as the soil rests in preparation for new life, we, too, can use this time to turn inward, heal, and prepare for the next growth cycle.

The power of winter in manifestation is not just symbolic; it is deeply rooted in how the mind and body function during this season. As the world outside quiets, our brains naturally enter a state of introspection and profound recalibration. This is a time to release what no longer serves us, reprogram limiting beliefs, and strengthen our subconscious alignment with our desires. Much like seeds buried beneath the snow, our manifestations are forming in unseen ways, preparing to emerge when the time is right.

Neurologically, winter provides the perfect conditions for profound transformation. During this season, we often experience lower levels of external stimulation, allowing greater focus on inner work. Meditation, journaling, and visualisation become even more powerful tools as they help us reshape our neural pathways and strengthen our beliefs about what is possible. This process is supported by melatonin, the hormone that regulates sleep and rest. With longer nights and reduced exposure to artificial stimulation, winter encourages us to enter a deeper, more restorative state where true transformation begins.

Although winter is a time of stillness, it is also a time of profound inner work. Just as nature trusts the unseen renewal process, we must trust that our desires align, even without immediate evidence. This season teaches us the power of surrender and patience - to embrace the quiet, trust the timing, and nurture our inner world to fully prepare when the time for action arrives.

Winter is more than just a pause between seasons; it is a sacred space for rest, healing, and alignment. By consciously working with its energy, we lay the foundation for powerful manifestations that will emerge in divine timing. Just as the earth quietly prepares for the bloom of spring, our dreams are taking shape beneath the surface, ready to unfold when the moment is right.

Winter Workbook

Winter is the season of rest, introspection, and renewal - a time to retreat inward, embrace stillness, and replenish your energy. While autumn is about letting go, winter invites you to trust the stillness, embrace deep reflection, and prepare for rebirth in spring. This is not a season of outward action but rather an inner transformation. Suppose you have been moving through the previous workbooks. In that case, you will be well established with the forward movement of setting intentions, aligning emotions, affirmations, visualisations, letting go and gratitude. Now is the time to refine your beliefs and align with your soul's more profound wisdom.

Revisit the Life Balance Wheel (page 96) and ask yourself: What do I need to nurture within myself right now? What dreams am I incubating? What fears or doubts still need to be cleared?

Winter is a time for intuitive guidance, journaling (page 108), and dream work (page 232). Explore subconscious reprogramming, deepen meditation practice, and reconnect with your inner wisdom. This is also the season for reflection, forgiveness, and self-love rituals. Meanwhile, manifestation requires trust, surrender, and alignment. Winter teaches us that sometimes, the most powerful thing we can do is pause, listen, and allow.

As you rest and recharge, prepare yourself for the new cycle ahead. Spring will bring fresh energy, new opportunities, and another chance to step forward in alignment with your highest self.

We start winter with the Winter Solstice in December and then have three full moons. In January, with the energy of 'Inner Reflection and Intuition', we have the 'Wolf Moon', named after the howling of wolves during winter. Then, in February, we have the 'Snow Moon' with the energy of 'Cleansing and Renewal' representing purity, renewal, and the quietude of winter. Then, finally, in March, with the energy of 'Rebirth and Growth', we have the 'Worm Moon', which signifies the emergence of earthworms as the ground thaws, symbolising 'Rebirth, Fertility, and the Awakening of Nature'. All of these have practical exercises and online meditations.

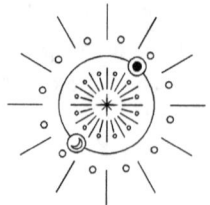

"You become what you believe."

Oprah Winfrey

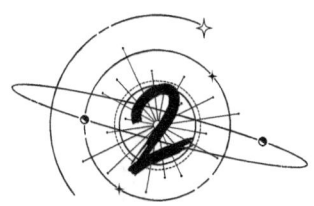

Review and Reflect

Other than just picking intentions out of thin air - generally based on your ego or something you feel is lacking within you when you compare yourself to others - I suggest taking a deeper dive into yourself and setting empowering, life-changing intentions that align with your soul purpose. This can involve shadow work (page 228) and overcoming trauma. But putting the inner work in and discovering the deep self is all part of the journey to clearing a path for meaningful change. This inner work should be done in winter when the Cosmic energy is aligned for inner reflection and transformation. You can use many tools and exercises to set your intentions on your manifestation journey, and I will hold your hand through this process using several tools in the winter and spring workbooks.

You may instinctively already know the intentions you wish to set or at least feel what you are missing from life or what you want to change. But I have found that people often do not honestly know and say, "I will be happy when XYZ." This is the completely wrong thing to do.

To help with this, I have included two life review exercises, which I do with all my classes: the Ikigai and the Life Balance Wheel. Once you have completed these, you will better understand where you are today and where your soul is trying to guide you. With this knowledge, you will be in a better place to set meaningful intentions. Based on where you are now and where you wish to get to.

Before you undertake the following exercises, ask yourself:
Do I know my soul's purpose?
Do I know where I am now?
Do I know what is missing?
Do I know what direction I am going?
Do I know what I want to manifest?
Do I know what intentions to set to achieve this?

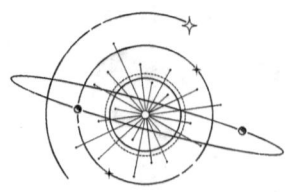

Ikigai - Soul Purpose

Ikigai is a Japanese concept that refers to a person's life purpose or reason for being. It is a way of finding joy and fulfilment by aligning your passions, talents, and profession with the world's needs. It comprises four interlocking circles, as shown below, in which you place the answers to a set of questions/reflections.

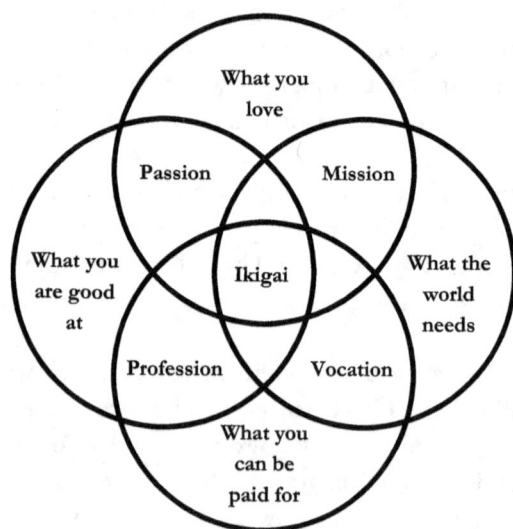

I have taught this for several years with profound results. I see faces light up as participants discover so much about themselves. One potent moment was when a tear rolled over the cheeks of a retired lady who put 'accomplished' in the Ikigai circle, with her realising she had not only found her 'Soul Purpose' but had 'Lived It'. It was such a beautiful moment. But she now uses this exercise for personal aspirations.

A full-size version is overleaf for you to complete, and if this is too small to complete, you can print out an A4 version on my website.

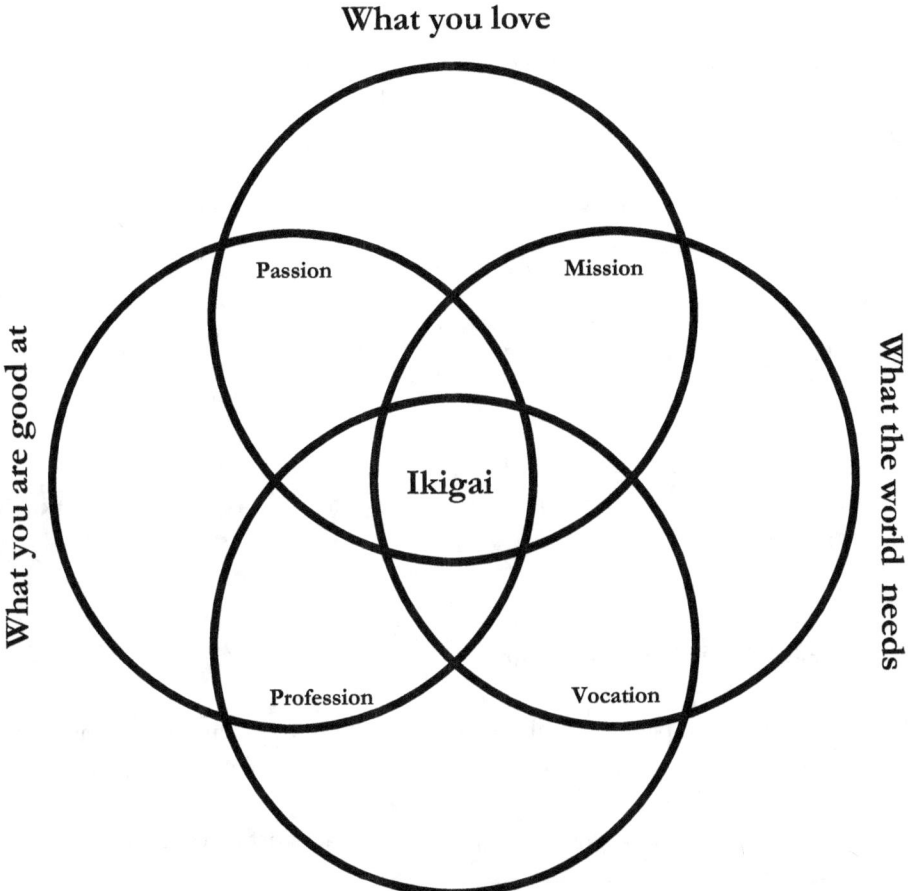

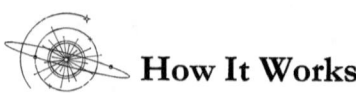 **How It Works**

1. In the circle on the left - 'What you are good at'

Write down your skills, talents, and unique abilities - the ones you were born with and the ones you learnt and mastered during your personal life, work, or education. Your existing skills, talents, and expertise are essential.

Ask yourself what you know well - everything you have done with good results until now has potential value.

Extra helpful questions to analyse:
- What do I excel at doing?
- Is there something I want to be among the best at with some more education and experience?
- Which parts of my (current and/or past) job am I good at?
- What am I among the best at within my school/workplace and/or community?

2. In the top circle - 'What you love'

Write things you are passionate about, activities that bring you joy, and tasks and topics that motivate you to get out of bed in the morning feeling excited.

You need to ask yourself what fascinates you, what satisfies you, and what you have the most fun doing.

Additional helpful questions to ask yourself:
- What is thrilling to me?
- What could I talk about for hours on end?
- What would I do if I did not have to be concerned about making money and getting paid?
- How would I spend my time on holiday or a free weekend?

3. In the circle on the right - 'What the world needs'

Note down what your potential clients/community would benefit from but is not accessible to them - or how you can do it better.

What you are offering has to be something needed in the world so you do not end up putting a lot of your precious time and energy into something nobody wants or needs. Analyse what the market needs that you can provide better than your competition (or at least that offers better value to begin with). Is there anything particular that your potential clients/community are trying to accomplish in their work or lives, and what tasks and problems do they want to solve?

Other questions to ask yourself:
- What issues in my community would I like to help solve?
- What matters in my community that I care about, and what problems affect me emotionally?
- Will some of my work be relevant a decade from now, and whose life will it influence?

4. In the bottom circle - 'What I can be paid for'
Write down services, tasks, and niches that may give you the most significant return on your time investment and for which you can get paid more.

We have to pay our bills, and no matter what, your Ikigai should not keep you up at night wondering how to stay afloat. It would be a shame to, at best, break even from a 'pricey hobby' that takes up your time, money, and emotional resources.

Some other important questions to ask yourself:
- For what work have I already been paid?
- Are other people being paid for this work?
- Am I already making a good living doing what I am doing?
- If not, according to the current market, can I eventually make a good living doing this work?
- Are people willing to pay for what I am doing/selling?

The 'Four Inner Eclipses'

Now, you can move to the inner eclipses and note anything that appears in <u>both</u> the bigger circles.

1. **Passion** - In this eclipse, write down anything that appears in <u>both</u> 'what you love' and 'what you are good at'.

2. **Mission** - In this eclipse, write down anything that appears in <u>both</u> 'what you love' and 'what the world needs'.

3. **Vocation** - In this eclipse, write down anything that appears in <u>both</u> 'what the world needs' and 'what you can get paid for.'

4. **Profession** - In this eclipse, write down anything that appears in <u>both</u> 'what you are good at' and 'what could make you money.'

**Now, look at all these four eclipses,
if anything repeats
in <u>ALL FOUR</u>
then you have your Ikigai**

Your Life Purpose

What if you cannot find your Ikigai

If you did not have anything in all four eclipses - where passion, mission, vocation, and profession overlap - it is entirely okay! It just means you need to explore further.

Here is what you can do:

Reflect on what is Missing
- Look at each of the four sections:
    - What you love
    - What you are good at
    - What the world needs
    - What you can be paid for
- Could you identify which section feels empty or weaker? That is where you need to focus.

Experiment and Explore
- Try new hobbies, volunteer, or take on different roles.
- Learn new skills or deepen existing ones.
- Talk to people in different careers or lifestyles that interest you.

Find Patterns in Your Life
- Think about activities that naturally excite you.
- Please remember past moments when you felt deeply engaged or fulfilled.
- Ask friends or mentors what they think you are great at.

Start with What You Have
- Could you work with that if only two or three sections are filled? For example, if you know what you love and are good at, explore ways to make it worthwhile to the world or monetise it.

Be Open to Change
- Ikigai is not something you find instantly - it evolves.
- Your centre might change as you grow and gain new experiences. Mine certainly did.

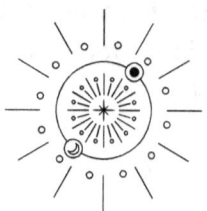

"Balance is not something you find, it is something you create."

Jana Kingsford

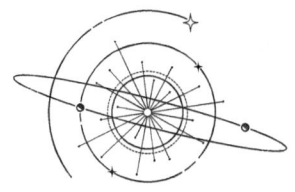

Life Balance Wheel

This is a powerful self-assessment tool used to evaluate different areas of your life and identify areas for improvement. It visually represents self-awareness and highlights the balance or imbalance across key life areas. Often highlighting areas where you may feel unfulfilled or off balance. Once identified, these areas can help you set meaningful goals and focus. It can also be used to track your progress over time.

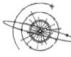 **How It Works**

The 'Life Balance Wheel' is typically a circle divided into segments, each representing a different aspect of life. You rate your satisfaction in each area on a scale from 1 to 10, then plot these scores on the wheel. The result shows whether your life feels balanced or areas that need attention. These out-of-balance areas are usually where your first manifestation intentions come from.

 Common Life Areas in a Life Balance Wheel

Though categories can be customised, a standard version often includes:

- Career and Work - Job satisfaction, growth, and fulfilment.
- Finances - Stability, income, and financial security.
- Health and Wellness - Physical and mental well-being.
- Personal Growth - Learning, self-improvement, and mindset.
- Relationships - Love, friendships, and family connections.
- Spirituality - Inner peace, faith, or connection to a higher purpose.
- Fun and Recreation - Hobbies, leisure, and joy.
- Environment - Living space, work environment, and surroundings.

If there is another area in your life you wish to track, replace one of the categories or add another slice to the pie - make it personal to you.

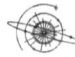**What to do**

- Consider each area of life and rate it on a scale of 1 - 10, with 1 being completely dissatisfied and 10 being completely content.

- Then, draw a line around the arc or colour in the section from the centre towards the appropriate arc.

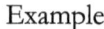

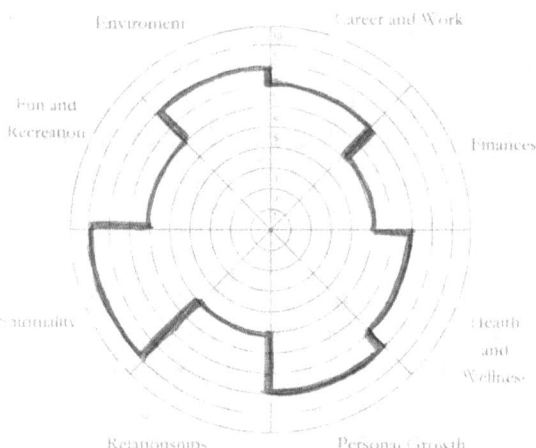

Most people first look to manifest those areas with a low score (closer to the centre) to bring life back into balance.

Compare the two tools to identify which aspects of your life may be unbalanced and how they align with your soul's purpose. Setting intentions in these areas would be beneficial.

— Life Balance Wheel —

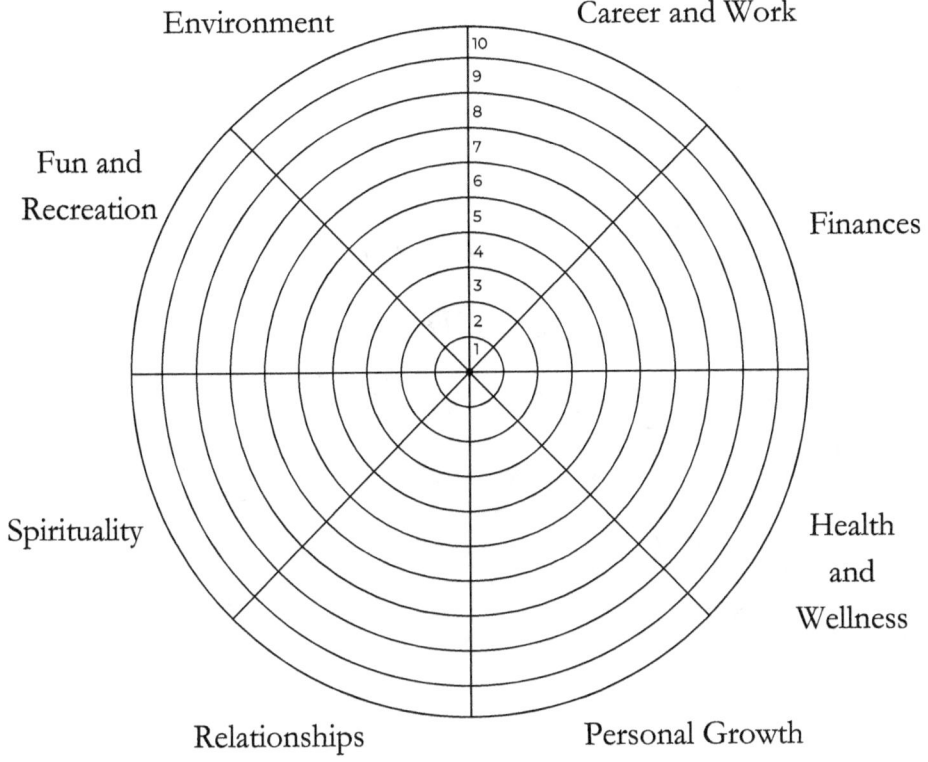

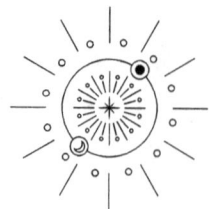

*"Your intentions
create
your reality."*

Wayne Dyer

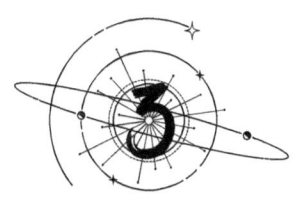

Set Your Intentions

"Intentions matter - what you send out, you receive back!"

Teanna

Manifestation involves several key aspects that combine to bring your desires into reality, the third step being - setting clear intentions. With this, there are only three rules to get the best outcome with intentions:

 Write them in the present tense
As if it has already happened. Do not create too many. I suggest starting with one long-term intention, one mid-term intention, and two short-term intentions.

 Be specific
Knowing precisely what you want is essential, as it focuses and directs your manifestation process. Let us take the example of desiring to manifest a new job. Do not be vague and wish for "a better job." Be specific, i.e., "I manifest a position as a marketing manager at a well-established company where I can apply my skills and grow professionally." Other examples are in the 'Setting Intentions Reference Guide', page 198.

 Keep the intention positive!
Set without ego and not aimed to harm anyone or anything. Negative examples can be found in the 'Setting Intentions Reference Guide'. Page 198.

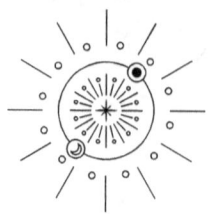

"When you are in alignment with the desires of your heart, things have a way of working out"

Iyanla Vanzant

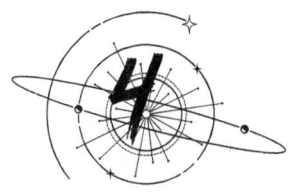

Emotional Connection

Now that you have your meaningful intentions, you need a way to evoke a positive feeling towards them - this is the key to manifesting - this is what programmes the mind to see the opportunities the Cosmos puts in front of you. Evoking emotional states can be done via several techniques, depending on how you are as a learner - written (journalling) and visualisation (meditation) are the two most common - but songs (writing your own or listening to others) and creativity (vision boards/painting) can also be used.

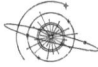**How This Fuels Manifestation**

The brain cannot distinguish between a real experience and a vividly imagined one. When you infuse your intentions with intense emotional energy, your brain (your RAS) begins to believe those experiences are already unfolding and draws your attention to the opportunities.

- Feeling genuine gratitude, joy, or excitement before something happens sends a powerful signal to your brain - it reacts as though the desire has already been fulfilled.

- Emotions act as amplifiers, reinforcing the neural pathways linked to your goals and aligning your mindset, behaviours, and energy with your desired reality.

- This emotional state then draws in people, opportunities, and experiences that reflect it.

The key is to embody the emotions of your future now - gratitude, love, joy, and excitement. These feelings signal to the Cosmos that your vision is real, drawing that future closer by aligning your energetic state with the reality you want to create.

So how do you do this?

The first thing you need to acknowledge is that we all learn differently, which should be reflected in the tools you choose to evoke emotions. For example, if you are an auditory learner, writing affirmations at great length each day will not evoke the emotions of pleasure, excitement and joy but will evoke feelings of frustration and boredom. An auditory learner will have much more success by listening to recorded affirmations to evoke the pleasure, excitement and joy emotions.

Here are the different learning styles. Which are you?

Visual learners - 65% of the population
They prefer to see information to understand and remember it. They often use charts, diagrams, mind maps, and colour-coded notes to help organise their thoughts. Watching videos, viewing demonstrations, and using visual aids can significantly enhance their learning experience. To evoke emotions, these learners will succeed more with 'sight-based' tools.

- Vision boards with emotionally charged images
- Visualisation practices (imagine scenes in vivid detail)
- Mind maps or mood boards for desires
- Watching inspiring videos or films that spark emotion
- Colour-coded affirmations or journaling
- Creative visual scripting (drawing out your future life)
- Watching your future self like a movie in your mind

Auditory learners - 30% of the population
They absorb information best through sound. They learn most effectively when they listen to instructions, engage in discussions, or hear concepts explained out loud. To evoke emotions, these learners will have more success with 'sound-based' tools.

- Spoken affirmations (with emotion)
- Voice notes or audio journaling
- Guided meditations with vivid language
- Binaural beats and solfeggio frequencies (e.g., 528 Hz, 432 Hz)
- Manifestation playlists or emotional music
- Talking through visualisations with a coach or friend
- Chanting or mantras

Kinaesthetic learners - 5% of the population
They learn best through physical activity and hands-on experience. They prefer actively participating in the learning process, whether building something, experimenting, or using movement to reinforce concepts. These learners often benefit from roleplaying, interactive tasks, or even walking around while studying. The more they can involve their body, the better they learn. To evoke emotions, these learners will succeed more with 'touch and movement-based' tools.

- Embodiment exercises ("act as if" - walk, talk, move like your future self)
- Dance or movement to music that evokes emotion
- Physically writing affirmations or scripting (pen to paper)
- Vision walks (visualising while walking or exercising)
- Creating rituals with physical objects (candles, crystals, symbolic items)
- Roleplaying or acting out your future scenarios
- Sensory anchoring (using smell, touch, and movement to lock in emotion)

Reading/writing learners - Often grouped under visual
They thrive through written words. They absorb information by reading textbooks, taking detailed notes, journaling, or rewriting ideas in their own words. These learners enjoy working with lists, essays, and written exercises and often prefer quiet, independent study time. To evoke emotions, these learners will succeed more with 'text-based' tools.

- Scripting your future in a journal (in present tense)
- Gratitude journaling with emotional depth
- Reading inspirational books, quotes, or stories
- Writing affirmations and repeating them
- Letter to your future self (or from your future self)
- Creating a manifestation journal or planner
- Reviewing written goals daily and reflecting on how they feel

Multimodal learner - 60–70% (overlap with others)
They combine two or more learning styles and switch between them depending on the task or subject. For example, someone might prefer reading to learn new material but find it easier to remember through discussion or drawing diagrams. Being multimodal allows for flexibility, and these learners often benefit from mixing techniques to keep their learning dynamic and engaging. To evoke emotions, these learners will have more success with a blend of styles - feel free to mix and match.

- Listen to your voice-recorded affirmations while journaling
- Create a vision board and describe it aloud
- Meditate while visualising and repeating mantras
- Script by hand, then read it aloud with feeling
- Dance to a manifestation playlist while visualising your desires

Once you have decided which type of learner you are - you can choose a selection of tools to help you evoke the desired emotions. If you do not know what type of learner you are - take the test on page 210

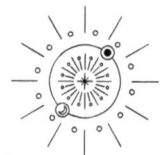

"Change begins with one thought, which becomes one feeling, which becomes one step - but persistence is what paves the way to transformation"

Teanna

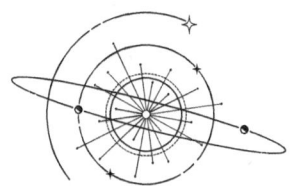

Visualisation

Visualisation is one of the most effective ways to evoke emotion for manifestation. This includes mental imagery (internal) and physical visual tools (external). In both cases, it is not simply about seeing your desired future but about truly feeling it - creating the intention as if it is already here.

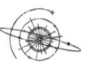 **Internal visualisation**

This imagination-based practice takes place entirely within your mind's eye. It involves mentally seeing, feeling, and experiencing your desired outcome as if it were now. Visualisation is often used during meditation, scripting, or quiet moments of reflection, where you intentionally create vivid mental scenes that align with your goals. Because your inner world entirely generates it, you can shape your vision in a deeply personal and emotionally resonant way.

What makes internal visualisation so powerful is its direct connection to the subconscious mind - the part of you responsible for your beliefs, habits, and automatic responses. By involving all your senses - sight, sound, touch, even smell and emotion - you create a full-bodied experience that your brain begins to accept as real. This emotional embodiment is key to reprogramming limiting beliefs and aligning your energy with what you want to attract.

For example, imagine closing your eyes and receiving a phone call telling you, you have landed your dream job. You hear the excitement in your voice, feel your heart race with joy, and picture the room around you as it all unfolds. At that moment, your body begins to respond as if it is already real - and that is when manifestation becomes genuinely magnetic.

> **TRY** Imagine the life you want as if it is unfolding right now, and involve all your senses in the experience. See the details, hear the sounds, smell the smells, taste the tastes, and feel the energy of the environment around you. Most importantly, connect with the emotions that would come with it - joy, freedom, peace, and gratitude.

Internal visualisation is compelling when practised just after waking or before sleep when the mind is most open and receptive. This simple yet transformative practice helps build a strong emotional connection to your goals, keeping you aligned and inspired. Visualising your success in rich, vivid detail creates a mental blueprint that draws in opportunities aligned with that vision. Just like a seed needs water, sunlight, and care to grow, your goals need the consistent nourishment of focused thought, aligned emotion, and intentional action.

However, some people struggle to visualise internally - this is called aphantasia. People with aphantasia can think about or describe things in detail, but they cannot see those images in their minds like most others do. It is not considered a disorder - just a different cognitive processing style. For example, if you close your eyes and try to picture a beach, someone with aphantasia may intellectually know what a beach looks like but will not experience a mental image of it.

The exact cause of aphantasia is not fully understood. Still, it is believed to be related to differences in brain connectivity, particularly between areas responsible for memory, visual processing, and imagination. It is often genetic and lifelong, although many people do not realise they have it until they discover that others can "see" vivid mental images.

Importantly, people with aphantasia can still manifest effectively. You do not need to visualise an image to manifest. What matters most is your ability to feel the emotion, hold the intention, and use other senses, such as sound, language, and physical sensation, to create internal alignment. Many aphantasics are excellent manifesters because they naturally lean on powerful alternatives like vision boards, scripting, auditory affirmations, and embodiment practices.

Your desired reality is far more critical than being able to see it. Manifestation does not depend on how you can visualise an image - it depends on how you believe in it and how deeply you feel it.

External visualisation

This is a physical, sensory-based practice in which your desires are represented through tangible tools you can see and interact with in your external environment. These tools include vision boards, printed photos, post-it note affirmations, Pinterest mood boards, or any visual representation of your goals. These tools are powerful reminders of what you are calling in, helping to trigger emotion, focus your intention, and keep your vision front of mind throughout the day.

External visualisation is so effective because it reinforces your desires visually, over and over again. Seeing your goals represented concretely and physically helps clarify and solidify what you genuinely want. It benefits people who are more visually oriented or thrive with regular reminders and cues in their space. For example, creating a vision board filled with images of your dream home, ideal lifestyle, travel goals, or empowering quotes and placing it somewhere you will see daily can keep you emotionally connected and energetically aligned with your future.

 ### Vision Board

Vision boards are popular for a reason, but do not just use them passively. When you look at your board, connect emotionally with each image. Feel the joy, excitement, or peace that achieving each goal would bring. That emotional heart energy sends a strong signal to the brain - and the Cosmos.

- Digitally, this can be done with apps like Pinterest or Canva and set as your phone wallpaper so you see it daily, as seeing it daily reminds your subconscious of your goals.
- Physically, this can be done on boards with magazines and printed cutouts. The hack, though, is to have it somewhere where you will see it daily to reinforce your vision.

 ### Creative Visualisation Through Art

If you are creative, draw, paint, or doodle your desires. If you are not an artist, sketch symbols or scenes representing your goal. The act of creating reinforces the vision.

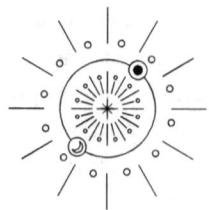

"The combination of your thoughts and feelings is your state of being. Change your state of being... and change your reality."

Dr. Joe Dispenza's

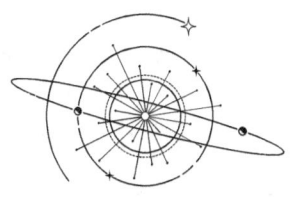

Journaling and Scripting

Journaling is a form of written visualisation and a powerful manifestation technique, especially if you process through writing or often have a busy mind. This method involves writing about your desired reality in the present tense as if it has already come true.

For example: "I am so grateful for the freedom I now have in my career." Let the emotion flow through your words - the more you feel what you write, the more deeply it embeds into your subconscious.

Describe your life in vivid detail within your manifestation: where you are, how you feel, what you are doing, and who you are with. Use positive affirmations and present-tense language to affirm that your desires are already unfolding. This brings clarity to your vision and strengthens the emotional connection needed to attract it into your reality. (See Page 172 for affirmation examples.)

While scripting and journaling can be incredibly powerful manifestation tools, they may not work equally well for everyone, especially if they lack emotional connection. Simply writing affirmations or desires without truly feeling them turns the practice into a mechanical task, which makes your subconscious mind less likely to respond or shift.

Another reason scripting may fail is that it keeps you stuck in your head rather than your heart or body. For some people, writing becomes a form of overthinking - trying to get the words "just right" instead of genuinely connecting with the vision. This mental overanalysis can block the emotional energy needed for manifestation to work.

It can also feel inauthentic or forced, especially if your writing statements do not yet feel believable. If saying "I am living my dream life" feels fake or creates inner resistance: your subconscious may reject the message - which can reinforce the feeling that it is untrue. Additionally, scripting and journaling may not resonate with those whose dominant learning style is not verbal or written. If you are more of a kinaesthetic, visual, or auditory learner, you may find it harder to evoke strong emotions through writing alone. In these cases, movement, sound, or imagery may be more effective tools for accessing that aligned emotional state.

Finally, it is essential to remember that journaling alone is not enough. While it can help align your energy and clarify your desires, it must be paired with inspired action. Writing is a supportive tool, not the entire process. Without follow-through or embodiment, journaling can become more of a wish list than a manifestation practice.

In short, scripting and journaling are most effective with genuine emotion, belief, and aligned energy. If they feel flat or disconnected, exploring other methods that better suit your style and emotional wiring is okay. If journaling does appeal, try:

 A Day in My Ideal Life
Write a complete journal entry describing one perfect day in your dream life - as if you are living it now. Use the present tense and include rich sensory and emotional detail. Focus on how you feel, what you are doing, who you are with, and what surrounds you.

Why it works
It activates your imagination and emotion, which helps impress the vision onto your subconscious mind.

Letter from Your Future Self
Purpose: To create self-belief, build confidence, and get guidance from the wiser, future version of you. Imagine yourself one year into the future, already living your desired life. Write a letter from that future version of you to your current self. Include encouragement, reminders, advice, and gratitude for the steps you are taking now.

Why it works
It shifts your perspective, activates hope and motivation, and bridges the gap between who you are now and who you are becoming.

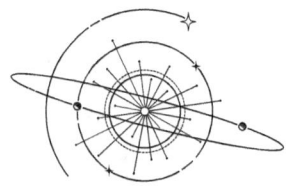

Embodiment

Begin to act as if your desired life is already yours. Imagine how your future version - the one who has already achieved the life you want - would walk, speak, make decisions, and carry themselves. Step into that energy now. By embodying the version of yourself who already lives that reality, you close the gap between where you are and where you are headed.

Align your daily habits, choices, and mindset with that vision. Speak, dress, and behave as if your goals are already unfolding. This signals to your subconscious that your desired reality is already in motion, creating internal alignment and attracting opportunities that reflect your new identity.

 Future - Self Visualisation

Imagine yourself five or ten years from now, having achieved your goals. Picture how you carry yourself, what you wear, who is around you, and how you feel. Step into the energy of that version of yourself.

 Movie Reel Method

Imagine your life as a movie where your intention has come true. Picture yourself as the main character, living your dream life. Play out scenes in your mind with confidence and excitement.

Make this a physical thing - use Canva and create a video by adding video shots of what you desire, then add upbeat music and watch the video every day.

To help with this, I have created a few, which can be found on my website or socials.

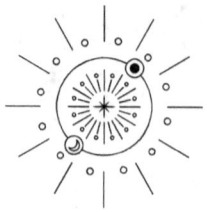

"When energy moves through sound and motion, intention becomes embodiment."

Unknown

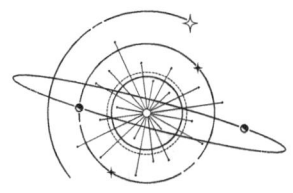

Sound and Movement

Music and movement can also trigger strong emotions. Moving your body and letting emotions flow helps shift your energy and amplifies your manifesting power.

 Playlists
Create a playlist with songs that empower, inspire, and energise you. Dance, sing, or listen and let the emotions rise.

 Meditation and Frequency Music
Listen to meditation music or frequency sounds (528 Hz for love, 432 Hz for healing, etc.). As you listen, close your eyes and picture your dream life. Let emotions flow naturally. The 'Sound Frequencies Reference Guide' on page 112 provides a list of suitable frequencies.

 Walking
Go for a walk and visualise your future self achieving your goals. Align your thoughts with your movements, feeling the success in every step. Nature walks enhance clarity and focus.

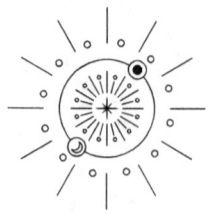

"Affirmations are the seeds of change - plant them daily, and watch your mindset bloom."

Unknown

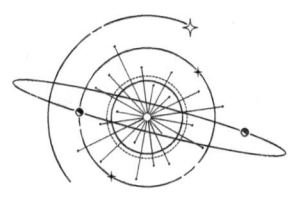

Affirmations

Affirmations are positive statements that help reprogram the subconscious mind by reinforcing beliefs, thoughts, and emotions that align with your desires/intentions. They are not just words you say out loud and expect magic to happen; they are words which need to evoke a 'feeling and emotion' - that is their job - to program your brain via feeling.

Affirmations are powerful because they help focus the mind on 'what is wanted' rather than 'lackin', allowing the energy of belief and expectation to shape reality. When repeated consistently and with feeling, affirmations strengthen neural pathways, making aligning with the frequency of your goals easier.

Individuals can cultivate a deep sense of self-worth and attract opportunities that match their intentions by speaking, writing, or visualising affirmations with conviction.

Affirmations should be personal to you, so I have provided many examples on page 172.

Affirmations can also help deepen your meditative experience by fostering a sense of balance and well-being. To take it deeper, you can use affirmations with the Chakra [2] energy centres by reciting the words to the corresponding centre (see page 214).

Affirmations can also be used to overcome limiting beliefs. I will walk you through this process in the Spring Workbook.

---

[2] Chakras are energy centers in the body, originating from ancient Indian spiritual traditions, particularly Hinduism and Buddhism. The word chakra means "wheel" in Sanskrit, and these energy points are believed to regulate the flow of life force energy (prana) throughout the body.

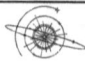 ## How Affirmations Work

Affirmations are powerful tools that influence our thought patterns and emotional states. We can shift our mindset and internal dialogue by repeating positive statements regularly. This mental shift can also impact the body's energy flow, helping to realign you with a more empowered emotional state. Over time, these affirmations can reprogram the subconscious mind, replacing limiting beliefs with more supportive and expansive ones.

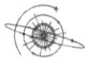 ## The Subconscious Mind – The True Manifestation Powerhouse

The subconscious controls around 95% of your thoughts, habits, and behaviours. It stores your deepest beliefs, emotional patterns, and memories - many of which were formed early in life and run automatically in the background. This makes it the true powerhouse of manifestation. If your subconscious holds limiting beliefs like "I am not good enough" or "I never get what I want," those hidden patterns can silently block your ability to manifest your desire.

However, when your subconscious beliefs are aligned with your intentions, manifestation becomes more natural and effortless. Techniques like hypnosis, scripting, deep meditation, and subliminal messaging can be used to access and reprogram the subconscious, clearing blocks and reinforcing new empowering beliefs.

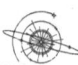 ## When and How to Use Affirmations

You can use affirmations at any time, but they are most effective when practised intentionally and consistently.

One of the best times to use affirmations is in the morning. Saying positive statements right after waking up helps set a good tone for the day. You can say them while looking in the mirror, during meditation, or while taking deep breaths. For example, you might say, "I am grounded, confident, and ready to embrace the day."

Another great time is before bed. Affirmations at night help calm the mind and reinforce self-love. You can say them while journaling, reflecting on your day, or even listening to recorded affirmations as you fall asleep. A good example is, "I am worthy of love and success. I release all worries and welcome peace."

Affirmations can also be helpful during stressful moments. When you are feeling anxious, overwhelmed, or experiencing self-doubt, repeating positive statements can help you regain control. This can be useful before a big meeting, presentation, or social events. A helpful affirmation might be, "I am in control of my thoughts and emotions. I choose peace over fear."

You can also use affirmations while exercising or doing yoga. This is a great way to boost confidence, motivation, and mindfulness. Saying things like, "My body is strong, my mind is focused, my energy is limitless," can help you stay aligned with your physical and mental well-being.

During meditation or visualisation, affirmations can help manifest specific intentions, such as love, abundance, confidence, or healing. They work well when combined with deep breathing or visualisation exercises. A powerful example is, "I attract abundance effortlessly. I am aligned with my highest self."

Affirmations are also helpful when facing challenges. Repeating positive statements can build confidence and resilience before an exam, job interview, or performance. They can also help during setbacks or when dealing with limiting beliefs. A helpful affirmation in these situations is, "I am capable. I trust my journey. Everything is working in my favour."

Finally, affirmations can be used throughout the day to reinforce positivity. Writing them on sticky notes, saying them while commuting, showering, or cooking, or setting them as phone reminders can help maintain a positive mindset. A simple but powerful affirmation is, "I radiate positivity and attract good energy."

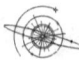 **How to use Affirmations with Number Frequencies**

Vortex Maths - Vortex math is a mathematical system based on patterns discovered by Marko Rodin. It focuses on repeating numerical cycles and the digital root of numbers, which means adding the digits of a number together until you get a single-digit result.

One of the core patterns in vortex math is the 1-2-4-8-7-5 cycle. When you continuously double numbers and reduce them to a single digit, they follow this sequence, which repeats infinitely. However, the numbers 3, 6, and 9 do not follow this pattern. Instead, they are considered divine numbers with special significance in energy and spirituality.

> *"If you only knew the magnificence of 3, 6, and 9, you would have the key to the universe."*
> — Nikola Tesla

Vortex math relates to affirmations because both are based on energy, repetition, and manifestation. Affirmations work by reprogramming the subconscious mind, and vortex math suggests that numbers have vibrational frequencies that can enhance this process.

One popular method that combines vortex math with affirmations is the 3-6-9 Affirmation Method. This technique involves repeating cycles 3, 6, and 9 affirmations to align with Cosmic energy. In this method, you:

- Say or write your affirmation 3 times in the morning to set your intention.
- Repeat it 6 times in the afternoon to amplify the energy.
- Say or write it 9 times at night to embed it into the subconscious.

For example, if your affirmation is "I am abundant and attract limitless opportunities," you would say or write it three times in the morning, six times in the afternoon, and nine times at night.

You can also apply vortex math to affirmations by structuring them around these powerful numbers. For instance, you can:

- Use three keywords to affirm: "I am powerful, confident, and successful." Repeat affirmations six times while meditating.

- Create a nine-word affirmation like: "I am in alignment with my highest purpose and joy."

Another way to integrate vortex math into affirmations is by using angel numbers and numerology[3], like 111, 222, or 333, which hold special energetic meanings. (A list of these can be found in the 'Repeated Numbers Reference Guide' on page 222)

You can enhance your affirmation practice by saying affirmations at 1:11, 2:22, or 3:33 PM or repeating affirmations 111 times over a period of days.

Another way is to choose affirmations that correspond to spirituality (3), love (6), and abundance (9).

Although vortex math is more philosophical and energetic than a scientifically proven principle, its focus on frequency, repetition, and patterns aligns with how affirmations work in the subconscious mind. The structured repetition of numbers helps reinforce neural pathways, increase belief in affirmations, and create a stronger, energetic imprint by reprogramming the subconscious mind and aligning your energy with your desires. Other methods include:

The 5x55 Manifestation Method

This method involves writing a chosen affirmation 55 times per day for five consecutive days while focusing on the feeling of already having what you desire. The repetition strengthens belief and sends a strong message to the subconscious mind.

---

(3) Numerology is the study of the mystical significance of numbers and how they influence our lives. Each number carries a specific vibration, energy, and meaning. Here are the most important numbers in numerology. See 'The Frequencies of Number Reference Guide'

For example, to attract financial abundance, you can write: "I am financially abundant, and money flows effortlessly to me." You would then write this statement 55 times every day for five days.

This method is effective because the number 5 represents change and transformation in numerology. Repeating the affirmation helps create momentum and reinforces one's belief in it.

The 33x3 Method

In this method, you write your affirmation 33 times daily for 3 days while visualising your goal as if it is already happening.

For example, if you are looking for a new job, your affirmation could be: "I am attracting my dream job effortlessly and joyfully." You would then write this statement 33 times per day for three days.

This technique is powerful because the number 3 symbolises creation and manifestation, while 33 is a master number in numerology associated with higher consciousness and spiritual awakening.

The 77x7 Method

The 77x7 method is similar to the previous ones but is used for long-term, life-changing goals. You choose an affirmation and write it 77 times per day for 7 days, focusing on gratitude and the feeling of already having what you desire.

For example, if you are manifesting love, you might write: "I am in a loving, fulfilling relationship with my soulmate."

This method works well because 77 is associated with intuition and enlightenment, making it ideal for profound subconscious transformation.

The Pillow Method

The pillow method is simple yet effective. You write your affirmation on a piece of paper and place it under your pillow before going to sleep.

Before sleeping, you read or repeat your affirmation and visualise your desire as if it has already come true. You can also repeat it in the morning upon waking.

For example, if your goal is happiness and success, your affirmation could be: "I am happy, successful, and living my dream life."

This method is effective because the subconscious mind is most receptive before sleep, allowing the affirmation to be absorbed deeply overnight.

 The Water Manifestation Method
This method uses water's energy to amplify affirmations. You begin by holding a glass of water and focusing on your affirmation. Then, you say the affirmation at least three times while visualising your desired outcome. Finally, you drink the water, believing that it is carrying the energy of your manifestation into your body.

For example, you might say: "This water is charged with positive energy. As I drink it, I attract success and happiness."

This technique is based on the idea that water can absorb and carry energy, as shown in Dr. Masaru Emoto's experiments on water and consciousness.

 The Mirror Method (Mirror Affirmations)
The mirror method involves standing in front of a mirror and saying affirmations out loud while looking at yourself. This helps reinforce self-belief and self-love.
For example, if you are working on confidence, you can say: "I am powerful, confident, and unstoppable."

Repeating affirmations in front of a mirror boosts self-perception and rewires the subconscious mind. It is particularly effective for confidence, self-love, and success.

 The 11:11 Method (Angel Number Manifestation)
The 11:11 method involves repeating your affirmation at 11:11 AM or PM or writing it 11 times daily. This is based on the belief that 11:11 is a powerful spiritual awakening number, often considered a portal for manifestation.

For example, an affirmation for alignment and abundance could be: "I am aligned with my highest purpose, and abundance flows effortlessly to me."

This method works well for those who believe in numerology, angel numbers, and spiritual synchronicities.

The Subliminal Affirmation Method

The subliminal affirmation method involves recording yourself repeating affirmations in a calm voice and listening to the recording while sleeping or meditating. This allows affirmations to bypass conscious resistance and go directly into the subconscious. For example, you can record: "I am successful, confident, and at peace with my life." Then, you listen to this recording every night before bed.

This technique is highly effective for changing deep-rooted beliefs, boosting confidence, and attracting abundance.

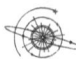 **Which Method is Best?**

The best method depends on your personal preference and the goal you want to manifest:

- **For Quick Results**
    - The 33x3 method
    - The Pillow Method

- **For Long-Term Transformation**
    - The 55x5 method
    - The 77x7 method

- **For Deep Subconscious Reprogramming**
    - The Subliminal Affirmation Method
    - The Water Manifestation Method

- **For Boosting Confidence and Self-Love**
    - The Mirror Method

- **For Spiritual Alignment**
    - The 11:11 method
    - The Vortex 3-6-9 method

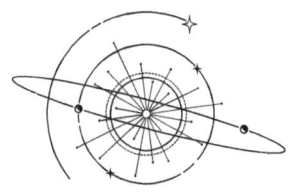

Gratitude

A daily gratitude practice can shift your emotional state almost instantly. By feeling thankful before your desires have physically arrived, you are training your brain and body to believe they already exist. Gratitude puts you in a state of abundance and trust, making it easier to attract what you want.

Before asking for what you want, acknowledge what you already have, as gratitude shifts your vibration from lack to abundance.

- Affirmations in the Present Tense: "I am so grateful for my thriving career" instead of "I hope to have a thriving career."
- Morning Gratitude List: Write down at least three things you are grateful for every morning.
- Gratitude Before Manifesting: Before visualising or affirming your desires, say, "I am so grateful for all I have and all that is on its way to me."
- Write a Gratitude Letter: Write a letter thanking the Cosmic Flow as if your manifestation has already happened.

 Use Gratitude in Visualisation

When visualising your desires, mentally express gratitude within the scene. Imagine yourself saying, "Thank you for this incredible opportunity!" or "I feel so blessed to live this life."

 Gratitude for Challenges

Even obstacles serve a purpose. Instead of resisting difficulties, say, "I am grateful for the lessons and growth this challenge brings me." This keeps your energy aligned with trust rather than fear.

 End the Day with Gratitude

Reflect on what went well each day, no matter how small. A nightly gratitude journal or saying "Thank you" before bed keeps your mind in a state of appreciation and openness.

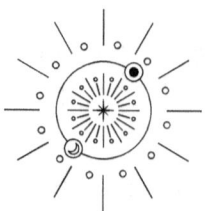

"Imagination is everything. It is the preview of life's coming attractions."

Albert Einstein

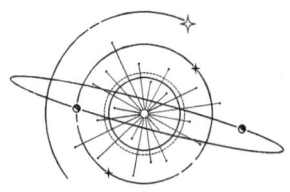

Meditation Techniques

Our fast-paced modern lives make it easy to feel overwhelmed by stress, scattered thoughts, and limiting beliefs that quietly pull us away from what we truly desire. Meditation offers a much-needed space of stillness - a moment to pause, breathe, and return to yourself. It allows you to escape the noise and reconnect with your intentions. When your mind becomes calm and centred, you naturally create the ideal mental and emotional environment to plant the seeds for the future you wish to create.

As explored in the 'Train Your Brain' chapter, one of the most transformative aspects of meditation is its ability to influence the subconscious mind. Most of our beliefs, patterns, and behaviours originate in this place, especially in the theta brainwave state (which occurs naturally in deep relation, after waking or before sleep); your mind becomes far more open and receptive. These are the golden moments to introduce empowering beliefs, vivid visualisations, and affirmations that align with the version of your life you are calling in.

Beyond stillness and clarity, meditation also helps you generate and amplify the emotional energy that fuels manifestation. Manifesting is not just about thinking about what you want but about embodying the feelings of already having it. Whether you focus on gratitude, joy, love, or abundance, meditation helps you connect deeply with those elevated emotions. These feelings shift your frequency, sending a clear message to the Cosmos about what you are ready to receive. The more consistently you align with these emotions, the more quickly your desires begin to form in reality.

There are numerous ways you can use meditation in manifesting:

Visualisation Meditation

Close your eyes and vividly imagine your desired reality. Picture it as if it is happening now, engaging all your senses and feeling its emotions.

 Future Self Meditation

Connect with the version of you who has already achieved your goal. Ask them questions, receive guidance, and embody their energy.

 Affirmation-Based Meditation

Repeat affirmations silently or aloud while in a meditative state. This helps anchor them more deeply into the subconscious mind.

 Scripting Meditation (Mental Scripting)

While meditating, mentally narrate your dream life as a story. Imagine speaking or journalling it as if it is already true.

 Gratitude Meditation

Focus solely on feelings of gratitude - both for what you have and for what you are calling in. Gratitude raises your vibration and draws in more of what you appreciate.

 Breathwork for Alignment

Use conscious breathing to regulate your nervous system and apparent resistance, creating space for intention-setting. Pair it with visualisation or affirmations.

 Theta State Meditation

Meditate when your brain is in theta state (right after waking or before sleep) to access your subconscious and embed new beliefs more easily.

Meditation Techniques

 Candle Manifestation Ritual

You can light a candle, look at the flame while visualising your intention, and speak your desire out loud with conviction.

 Energy and Chakra Work

Visualise energy flowing through your body, focusing on areas related to your intention. For example, if manifesting love, focus on the heart Chakra - pink light. If you desire financial abundance, focus on the solar plexus - yellow light. The heart chakra is also used for healing, but the green light is used. For spiritual growth, the crown Chakra and purple light are used. This aligns your energy with your manifestation. Please look at the 'Meditation and Chakra Reference Guide' on page 214 for details on the Chakra Centres.

 Emotion-Evoking Meditation

Focus entirely on cultivating emotions like joy, love, freedom, or abundance - the feelings you associate with your desired life.

 Body Scan with Intention

During a body scan, imagine energy flowing through each part of your body, clearing resistance and aligning you with your goals.

 Silent Meditation for Clarity

Sometimes, sitting in silence allows intuitive messages or inspired ideas to rise. This is great for clarity and receiving inner guidance.

 Third Eye Focus Meditation

Bring awareness to the space between your eyebrows and visualise your manifestation flowing through that channel. This practice is often used to strengthen inner vision and intuition.

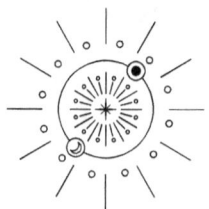

"Through meditation, we tune our inner frequency to the rhythm of the cosmos, where silence speaks and the universe listens."

Unknown

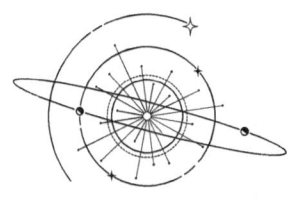

Cosmic Flow Meditation

This meditation can be found on www.TeannaTaylor.com called 'Unlock Your Cosmic Flow - Align to Cosmic Energy'

 Prepare for Deep Cosmic Flow Meditation

Time: 60 minutes

Online: Deep Cosmic Flow Meditation

Goal: Shift your brainwaves into theta and link with Cosmic energy to visualise your goals and rewire your brain

Steps: This is a five-part practice:

- Mindfulness (5 minutes)
- Body Relaxation (10 minutes)
- Disconnecting from Identity (15 minutes)
- Connecting to Cosmic Flow (10 minutes)
- Visualising the Goal (20 minutes)

How to Do It
- 1 Mindfulness
    - First, please decide what object to use for your mindfulness practice, such as a warm drink, a flower, or a candle.
    - Find a quiet place where you will not be disturbed
    - Sit in a comfortable position, and take some deep breaths, in through your nose and out through your mouth - big sigh breaths and feel your shoulders relax

- Focus all of your attention on the object in hand - use all of your senses
    - What do you see?
    - What do you feel?
    - What do you hear?
    - What do you smell?
    - What do you taste?

- Engage and get lost in the item.

This process relaxes the body and brings you into the present moment. It starts to slow your brain waves down and moves you out of Beta waves.

2 Body Relaxation
- When you feel relaxed, lie down (if you wish), close your eyes, and focus on your body.
- Slowly relax each part, going from top to bottom or bottom to top. If you do not feel relaxed and still have 'Monkey Mind'[4] thoughts coming in, do it again.

This process brings you down further into Alpha waves and will help to stop the monkey mind thoughts from popping up. If they do, 'give them to your monkey'(see page 63 for details on this)

3 Detach from Your Identity - Becoming No-Body
- Disconnect from your physical self. Imagine your body dissolving into pure energy as if floating in a vast, infinite space.
- Disconnect from past experiences and limiting beliefs
- As you meditate, let go of your name, roles, history, and problems, entering a state of pure awareness - where you are nobody, no one, in no time or place.

---

(4) Intrusive thoughts in meditation are unwanted, involuntary thoughts that disrupt focus and can be distracting, repetitive, or even distressing. They often take the form of random memories, worries, negative self-talk, or irrational fears. These thoughts arise because the mind naturally seeks stimulation, and unconscious thoughts surface when meditation slows mental activity. Stress and anxiety can also make them more frequent.

This process helps you detach from old mental patterns and become open to new possibilities. It activates your subconscious mind, which is crucial for rewiring your reality and enables you to detach from limiting beliefs.

4 Tune into the Cosmic Flow - Pure Consciousness
- Feel yourself connecting to an infinite field of possibility - this is the Cosmic flow.
- Begin to sense the energy around you.
- Imagine expanding beyond your body into an infinite energy field where everything is connected.
- Feel yourself merging with this space, becoming part of the vast intelligence that governs the Cosmos.

This step helps you detach from your current reality and shift into a new one.

5 Visualisation of Goals
- Imagine your goal unfolding step by step. Engage all of your senses:
  - What do you see?
    - Your ideal future is playing out, and your dream life is unfolding.

  - What do you hear?
    - People are congratulating you, and there are joyful sounds/nature sounds.

  - What do you feel?
    - Gratitude, excitement, fulfilment, joy, love

  - What do you smell/taste?
    - The fresh air of a dream location, a delicious meal.

  - Most importantly, FEEL the emotions of already having it.
    - If you are manifesting health, feel the vibrancy in your body. If it is financial abundance, feel the freedom and security.

- When ready, return to the room slowly, moving your toes or fingers
  - Place your hands over your eyes and open them into your palms
  - Do not rush; take it very slowly
  - Drink water
  - And feel the energy change inside you

By consistently practising this Cosmic Flow meditation, you align your energy with your desired future, reprogram your subconscious brain, and become a new version of yourself. Whether your goal is healing, financial success, love, or happiness, this practice helps bridge the gap between imagination and manifestation.

This meditation can be found on
www.TeannaTaylor.com called
'Unlock Your Cosmic Flow - Align to Cosmic Energy'

Transformation does not happen overnight. I encourage you to continue practising this meditation daily until your new thoughts, emotions, and energy become your default state. Over time, your brain rewires, and your external reality shifts to match your internal state.

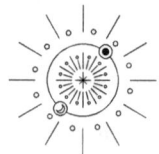

"Meditation is not about becoming a different person. It is about becoming the best version of yourself by quieting the noise and listening to your soul."

Teanna

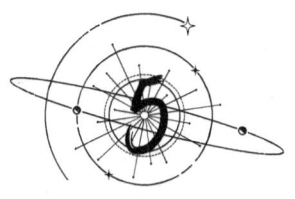

Trust and Flow

'Trust' is surrender, which means letting go of control, doubt, and attachment to how or when your desires will materialise. It is about trusting the Cosmos, allowing things to unfold naturally, and releasing resistance.

Surrender is essential because it removes resistance, aligns you with divine timing, shifts your mindset from lack to abundance, and creates inner peace, yet many people struggle with surrender because they try to micromanage their manifestations or worry about when they will happen. It is not about giving up but about allowing the Cosmos to bring you what is meant for you at the perfect time. However, true manifestation requires a balance between setting clear intentions, taking aligned action and then 'Flowing', i.e. allowing space for the Cosmos energy to work in its way but staying present and remaining open to signs from the Cosmos when it does via synchronicities.

Cultivating gratitude and acting as if your manifestation is already on its way can reinforce trust.

 Time: 5 minutes
Goal: Release resistance and trust the Cosmos to arrange the details.

How to Do It
Once you have established visualisations and affirmations to a point where you can evoke the feeling - allow it to heighten, and when you have reached a heightened emotional state, release attachment to the outcome. Say to yourself:

> "I surrender this to the Cosmos.
> I trust that everything is unfolding perfectly."

Feel light, open, and at ease - you are now flowing with the Cosmos, not forcing it. Let go of the "how" and "when" - trust that the energy flows and aligns events. Do not worry about how or when it will happen. Trust that the Cosmos is already working to rearrange reality in alignment with your new energy. Stay open to signs, synchronicities, and unexpected opportunities.

Why This Works
If you obsess over how something will happen, you create resistance. Surrendering allows the Cosmic Flow to work without interference.

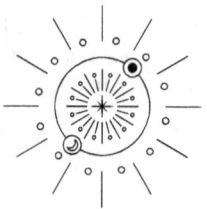

"What you think, you become.
What you feel, you attract.
What you imagine,
you create."

Buddha

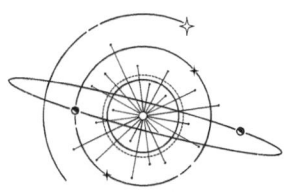

Synchronicities, Opportunities and Intuition

Synchronicities are meaningful coincidences that seem too perfectly timed to be random. Coined by psychologist Carl Jung, the term refers to events connected by meaning rather than cause and effect. These moments often feel like signs guiding you towards something significant. Examples include thinking of a friend you have not spoken to in years and suddenly receiving a message from them, frequently seeing repeating numbers like 111 or 222 when making important decisions, or coming across a book, quote, or song that perfectly relates to your current situation. I have listed the meaning of the repeated numbers in the 'Repeat Numbers Reference guide' on page 222.

Synchronicities are signs from the Cosmos offering guidance and confirmation that you are on the right path. To attract more synchronicities, it helps to stay present, set clear intentions, follow your intuition, and trust the process rather than forcing connections. These experiences remind us that life is interconnected and unfolding as it should.

Time: Ongoing (Daily Awareness Practice)
Goal: Recognise signs and take aligned action without force.

How to Do It:
- Pay attention to 'coincidences' and 'synchronicities' throughout the day - signs of the Cosmic Flow responding.
- Notice opportunities, unexpected messages, or intuitive feelings nudging you toward inspired action.
- Follow your gut instincts and act when something feels naturally aligned.
- Stay in a high-vibrational state - if you feel frustrated or impatient, return to gratitude.

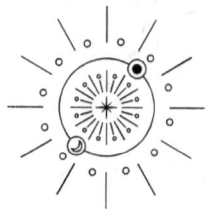

"Synchronicity is an ever - present reality for those who have eyes to see."

Carl Jung

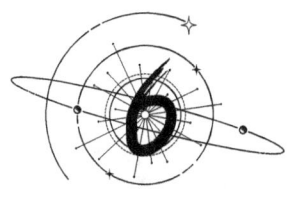

Inspired Action

Manifestation requires patience and a willingness to accept what comes, even if it differs from what you originally envisioned. While thoughts and feelings are powerful, manifestation often requires more than just thinking about your goal; it involves actively participating in its creation.

Aligned action means taking real-world steps that move you toward your goal while trusting that the Cosmos will guide you. Instead of just thinking about what you want, you must take intentional steps that bring your manifestation closer to reality. For example, if you are manifesting money, you can take action by looking for new income sources, applying for jobs, or offering a service. If your goal is to manifest love, you can be open to meeting new people, work on self-love, or update your dating profile. Similarly, if you are manifesting success, you might take courses, network with the right people, or start small projects that align with your goals.

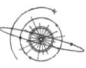 Follow the 'Next Right Step' Approach

You do not need to know every single step to achieve your goal. Instead, focus on taking one action at a time, trusting that the Cosmos will reveal the next step when the time is right.

A great way to guide your actions is by asking yourself:

"What is one thing I can do today that aligns with my manifestation?"

For example, if you are manifesting a business, you can start by researching your niche or creating a website. If your goal is better health, begin by drinking more water or exercising for just 10 minutes. If you are manifesting your dream home, you might start looking at listings or declutter your current space to make room for new opportunities.

By consistently taking small, aligned steps, you create momentum and signal your RAS to become aware of what the Cosmos puts in front of you.

Taking purposeful steps toward your goal shows your commitment and increases the likelihood of success. But the signs will be there. Be open to opportunities, remain flexible, and trust the process without being overly attached to the outcome; this allows you to flow with the natural course of events.

Time: Daily Habit
Goal: Embody your future self 'Now' to accelerate the manifestation.

How To Do It
Move, think, and act as if your manifestation is already unfolding. For example, if you manifest confidence, start walking, talking, and thinking confidently today. If you are manifesting financial success, start feeling abundant now, even if your bank account has not changed yet.

Remember, emotions like gratitude are key - express thankfulness daily for your future self.

Why This Works
When you align your actions and emotions with your desired future, you collapse time and bring it into your present faster.

Create a Mind Map
Time: 20 - 60 mins
Goal: Create a plan of action which is fluid and can be added to as opportunities arise

How To Do It
- To create a mind map, start with a circle in the centre of the paper - this is your overall goal.
- Then, draw sub-branches off and clearly label them.
- Then, draw sub-branches off that and break it down into smaller ideas, categories, or related concepts.
- Use colours, symbols, or images to clarify connections and enhance memory retention.
- Keep the structure flexible, allowing new ideas to be added as they arise.
- This visual approach helps organise thoughts, making complex information easier to understand and recall.

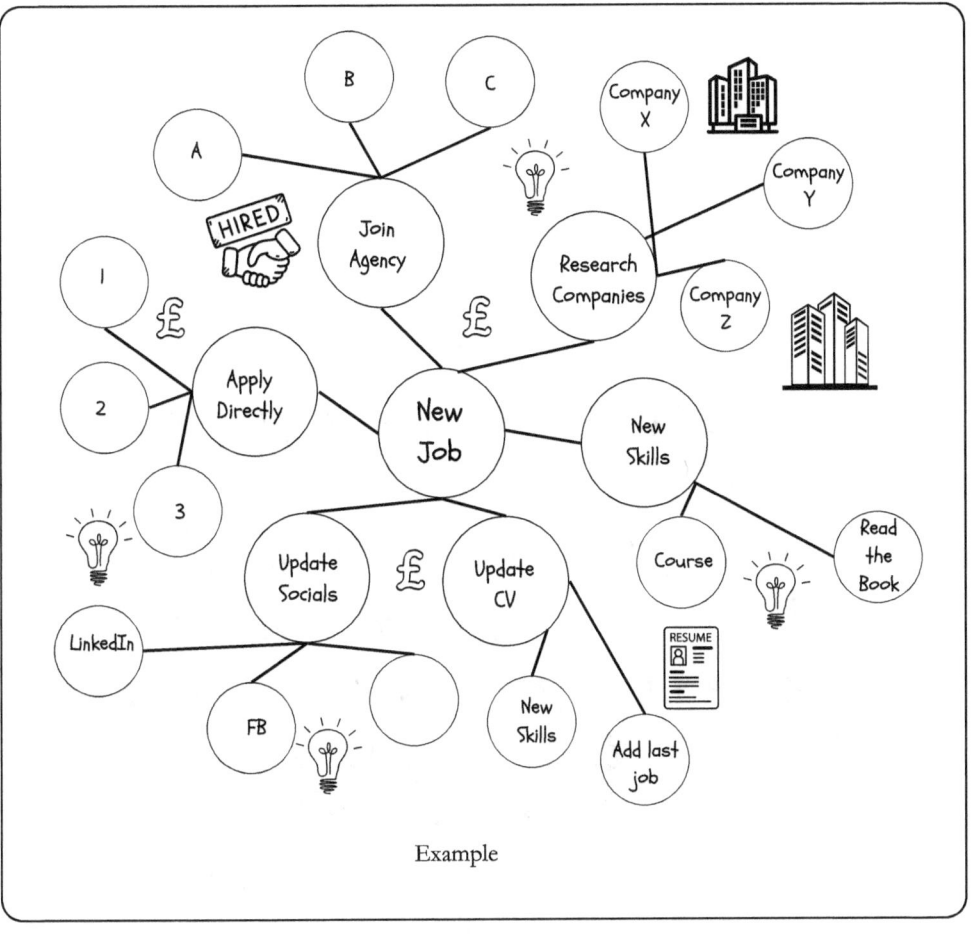

Example

Why This Works
Studies on goal-setting theory suggest that breaking larger resolutions into smaller, realistic steps increases dopamine (the brain's reward chemical), reinforcing positive behaviour and making it easier to stick to new habits.

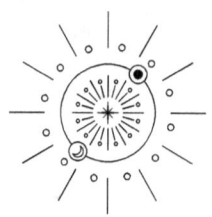

*"Remember
You Are the
Creator of Your Reality*

*The Cosmic Flow method
is a powerful blend of intentional
manifestation and cosmic surrender.
It teaches you to program your brain
for success, shift
your energy into alignment,
and then trust the
Cosmos to do the rest.*

*If practiced consistently, this method can
lead to profound transformations,
synchronicities, and unexpected
breakthroughs"*

Teanna

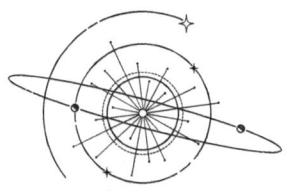

Putting It all Together

Here is a recap this is the six steps you have just learnt:

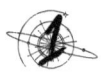 **Align yourself with the natural flow of the seasonal energies**

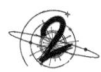 **Review and Reflect**

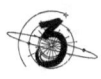 **Set Your Intentions**

 Emotional Alignment

 Trust and Flow

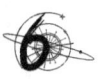 **Inspired Action**

Now that you have learnt the six steps, you need to remember that manifestation is a journey that unfolds in harmony with the natural cycles of the seasons, each phase playing a vital role in the process of creating, refining, and receiving.

And whilst you can manifest short-term goals anytime, i.e. finding a car parking space, big life-changing ones should have a daily routine that changes each season. This is so important as it is this where many fail to achieve their big life-changing dreams - remember, Spring is the season of planting seeds, setting intentions, and taking inspired action toward your dreams. As energy rises in summer, you step fully into embodiment and momentum, nurturing your manifestations with confidence and commitment. Autumn invites reflection, refinement, and release, allowing you to assess your progress and let go of what no longer serves you. Finally, winter is a time of stillness, deep alignment, and subconscious transformation - where your manifestations continue to take shape beneath the surface, preparing for their next evolution. By integrating these seasonal energies into your daily life, you create a powerful, natural rhythm that aligns you with the flow of the Cosmos, allowing manifestations to unfold effortlessly, in divine timing, and with deep trust in the process.

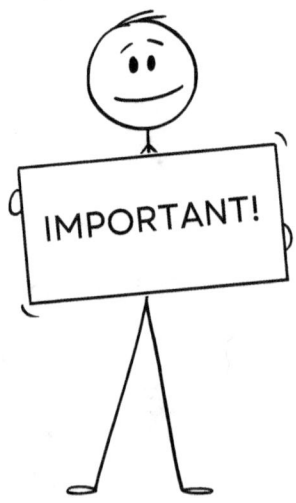

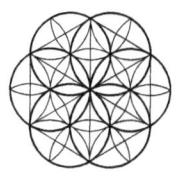

Daily Routine Spring

Spring is a season of renewal, fresh energy, and inspired action. It is when nature awakens from winter's stillness, and new growth begins. As seeds sprout and flowers bloom, we are called to set intentions, take bold steps forward, and embrace new opportunities. This daily spring manifestation routine will help you align with the energy of renewal, clarity, and expansion so you can step into your manifestations with confidence and purpose.

Morning Routine
Awakening Gratitude (5-10 min)
Step outside or open a window to breathe in the fresh spring air.
Feel the energy of renewal in the world around you.
Place your hand on your heart and say:
**"I welcome new beginnings.
I embrace fresh opportunities and step into my highest self."**

Spring Visualisation and Intention Journaling (10 min)
Imagine your dream life blossoming like the flowers around you.
Write down:
One new intention for the season.
One aligned action you will take today.
Three things you are grateful for in this moment.

Energising Movement (optional, 10 min)
Engage in gentle stretching, yoga, or a
morning walk to awaken your body.
Movement clears stagnant energy and opens space for new manifestations.

Midday

Spring-Inspired Affirmations (5 min)

Speak or write your personal affirmations that reinforce growth,
confidence, and abundance.
Finish with:
**"I am open to new possibilities.
Every step I take moves me closer to my dreams."**

Aligned Action Steps (10-20 min)

Spring is about momentum - take one inspired action toward your goal today.
Whether starting a new project, reaching out to someone,
or making a decision - small steps lead to significant results.

Connection with Nature (Varies by Day)

Spend time in nature to recharge and align with renewal energy.
For example, walk barefoot in the grass (earthing),
sit under a tree, or listen to birdsong.

Evening

Reflection and Gratitude (5-10 min)

Write down:
One small success from today.
One way you embraced new energy.
One thing you will release to make room for more growth.

Check in on your weekly task in the
Spring Workbook - Sow Seeds of Success (optional)

Nighttime

Visualisation and Spring Energy Meditation (10 min)
Before bed, visualise yourself thriving in your manifestations.
Use breathwork or guided meditation to clear any lingering doubts and
reinforce your belief in new possibilities.
Repeat: **"I am growing, expanding,
and stepping into my highest timeline."**

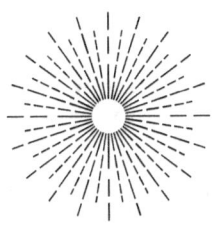

Daily Routine Summer

Summer is a season of momentum, confidence, and expansion, making it the perfect time to step into the full embodiment of your manifestations. This is the time for bold action, joyful celebration, and aligning with the high-energy frequency of the season. The sun's energy fuels momentum, and by aligning your daily actions, mindset, and rituals, you allow your manifestations to flourish and expand effortlessly. Live boldly. Take action. Manifest with power.

Morning Routine
Activate Your Energy and Intention (5 min)
On waking - Gratitude and Solar Connection
Step outside and face the sun (or Visualise its golden light).
Place your hand over your heart and take deep, energising breaths.
Express gratitude for your life, body, and the opportunities ahead.
**Say aloud: "I welcome the energy of the sun.
I step into confidence, expansion, and bold action today."**

Summer Visualisation and Embodiment (5 - 10 min)
Close your eyes and visualise your manifestations as already achieved.
Feel the emotions of success, joy, and abundance in your body.
Walk around your space acting as if you already have your desires.

Morning Action Plan (5 min)
Review your aligned action plan.
Choose one bold action for the day and commit to it.
**Write: "Today, I take inspired action toward [goal].
The Cosmos supports me."**

Midday
Embody and Align with Manifestation Energy
High-Energy Activity (20-30 min)

Move your body to activate vitality and flow (yoga, dancing, walking in nature).
Engage in activities that boost confidence and solar energy,
such as sunbathing, swimming, or outdoor grounding.
Even a walk outside will help.

Dopamine-Boosting Visualisation (5 min)

Take a moment to reflect on how your goals are progressing.
Use the Pomodoro Technique to stay focused on your tasks.

**Repeat: "Momentum is on my side.
I am unstoppable in my expansion."**

Manifestation Affirmations (optional)

Say or write affirmations that reinforce your bold, confident energy.
Example: "I am thriving in abundance. My dreams unfold effortlessly."

Evening
Reflection, Celebration and Moon Energy (5-10 min)

Sunset Reflection and Gratitude
Sit outside and watch the sunset, connecting with the energy
of completion and fulfilment.

Reflect on

What aligned action did I take today?
What synchronicities did I notice?
How did I embody my highest self?
Write down one success and celebrate it!

Check in on your weekly task in the
Summer Workbook - Cultivate Your Dreams (optional)

Nighttime
Body Relaxation and Wind Down Meditation (10-15 min)

Close the day with a body relaxation meditation to absorb the day's energy.
Visualise your manifestations coming to fruition effortlessly.
Set an intention for the next day with excitement and trust.

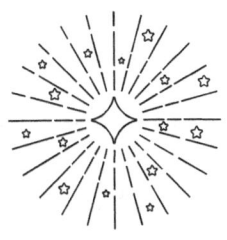

Daily Routine Autumn

Autumn is a season of introspection, transformation, and release - a time to gather the rewards of your efforts, let go of what no longer aligns with your path, and refocus on your highest vision. As trees gracefully shed their leaves to make way for new growth, this season invites you to clear space, reassess your journey, and prepare for fresh opportunities.

By embracing self-reflection, refinement, and release, you create the energetic space for new manifestations to take root. This is a time to honour your progress, trust the cycles of change, and step into the next phase of your journey with clarity and gratitude. The daily routine below will help you align with the natural rhythm of autumn, allowing you to manifest with intention, wisdom, and ease.

Morning Routine
Morning Journaling and Reassessment (10 min)
Use this time to check in with yourself and write freely.

Grounding and Gratitude (5-10 min)
Step outside or sit by a window and breathe in the crisp autumn air.
Place your hand on your heart and reflect on
what you are grateful for this season.
**Say aloud: "I honour the process of change.
I embrace reflection, release, and realignment."**

Seasonal Visualisation and Affirmations (5 min)
Picture yourself releasing what no longer serves you,
like trees letting go of their leaves.
Imagine your energy clearing and making space for what is to come.
**Repeat affirmations: "I trust the process.
I release with grace. I realign with my highest self."**

Taking Aligned Action (5 min)
Autumn is also a season of refinement - take one small, intentional step toward your manifestations.

Follow synchronicities and remain open to new directions and opportunities.

Evening
Evening Reflection (5-10 min)
Light a candle and reflect on the progress you have made.
Write down:
One thing I am proud of today
One lesson I learned
One thing I am grateful for

Check in on your weekly task in the
Autumn Workbook - Refine your Vision (optional)

Nighttime
Practice body relaxation meditation to release tension and align with the slowing rhythm of nature.
Visualise your manifestations integrating
effortlessly, knowing the Cosmos is working in divine timing.

Close your day with the affirmation:
"I trust the cycles of life.
I release with love and welcome what is meant for me."

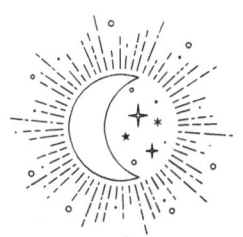

Daily Routine Winter

Winter is a season of stillness, introspection, and renewal. It is a time to turn inward, replenish your energy, and strengthen your connection to your deepest desires. Just as nature slows down to restore itself, this is your opportunity to pause, reflect, and realign before the growth cycle begins again in spring. Below is a daily winter manifestation routine designed to help you embrace the quiet power of this season while nurturing your manifestations in a gentle, aligned way.

Morning Routine
Slow and Mindful Wake-Up (5 min)

Instead of rushing out of bed, take a few deep breaths
and feel gratitude for the stillness of winter.
Place your hand over your heart and ask: What do I need most today?

Morning Reflection and Intention Journaling (10 min)

If you can remember your dream, make notes
Then, write down:
One thing you are grateful for.
One thing you are releasing.
One small, aligned intention for the day.

Gentle Winter Visualisation (5-10 min)

Imagine your manifestations as seeds resting beneath the snow, preparing for their perfect moment to bloom.
Feel deep trust in divine timing and repeat affirmations such as:
**"Everything is unfolding in perfect harmony.
I allow myself to rest, trust, and receive."**

Midday
Restorative Practices - Practice Mindfulness (5-10 mins)
Sip a warm drink and reflect on what your body and soul need.

Evening
Reflection and Gratitude (5-10 min)
Light a candle to symbolise inner warmth and clarity.
Spend time in quiet solitude, embracing the peace of the season.

Write down:
One thing you learned today.
One thing you are grateful for.
One thing you will release before sleep.

Small Acts of Self-Care and Restoration
Choose a different small act of self-care each night.
Examples include:
Take a warm bath with essential oils.
Read a book.
Engage in a hobby you enjoy.
Spend time with friends.
Have a massage.
Meditate. etc

Check in on your weekly task in the
Winter Workbook - Align Inner Transformations (optional)

Nighttime
Visualisation and Dream Incubation (10 min)
Before bed, visualise your future self thriving
in alignment with your desires.
Set an intention to receive guidance through dreams.
**Repeat affirmations such as: "I trust in the unseen.
My dreams are manifesting beneath the surface."**

Listen to a guided meditation (Optional)

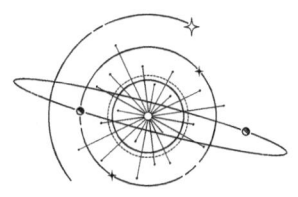

Real Life Examples

Other than my personal experience of overcoming a minor stroke and chronic illness, there are other reports of how this has worked for other people:

Career Advancement through Visualisation
Kristi Anderson, an independent nurse contractor, recounted when she sought a new job opportunity with better pay. After meditating and clearly articulating her desires, she was unexpectedly contacted by a former colleague offering her a position that matched her specified criteria. This experience reinforced her belief in the power of manifestation.

Personal Growth and Relationship Building
A contributor to the "Manifesting Success Stories" podcast shared her journey of personal transformation. By focusing on self-improvement and aligning her actions with her intentions, she experienced significant positive changes in her life, including improved relationships and a heightened sense of fulfilment.

Achieving Specific Personal Goals
Sabrina Carpenter, a well-known artist, revealed that she wrote her hit song "Espresso" as a "manifestation tactic" when she felt a lack of romantic interest in her life. The song's success, including topping the charts and amassing over a billion Spotify streams, exemplifies how she used creative expression as a form of manifestation to influence her personal and professional life.

For those interested in exploring more personal accounts of manifestation, the "Manifestation Success Stories" playlist offers a collection of experiences shared by individuals who have applied these principles in various aspects of their lives.

Oprah Winfrey
The media mogul has often discussed how her positive thinking and visualisations have significantly impacted her success. She believes that the energy we emit attracts similar energy back to us.

Jim Carrey
The actor and comedian famously wrote himself a check for $10 million for "acting services rendered" and dated it five years into the future. He kept the check in his wallet as a reminder of his goal. Just before the date he had written, Carrey received a role that paid him exactly $10 million.

Lady Gaga
The pop star has spoken about using mantras and visualisation techniques to manifest her success. Before achieving global fame, she repeatedly told herself she was a famous musician.

Arnold Schwarzenegger
Before achieving fame, Schwarzenegger used visualisation techniques to imagine himself as a successful bodybuilder and actor. He credits these mental practices as a significant factor in his achievements.

Denzel Washington
The acclaimed actor has mentioned his belief in the Law of Attraction, stating that you attract not only what you fear but also what you feel and are passionate about.

These individuals highlight the potential impact of positive thinking and visualisation in achieving goals.

Conor McGregor
The MMA fighter has spoken many times about visualising his victories before they happened:

"If you can see it here and have the courage to speak it, it will happen."

He claims that mentally rehearsing his wins and staying aligned with his goals helped bring them into reality.

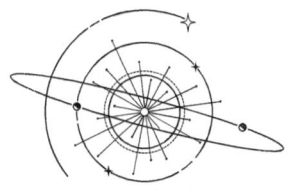

Cosmic Flow as a way of Life

Rather than something you do occasionally, manifesting can become a mindset, a way of interacting with the world, and a deep trust in the Cosmic flow of creation. When you live in alignment with manifestation principles, you naturally attract what you need, cultivate inner peace, and flow with life instead of resisting it. It transforms from a technique into a state of being where your energy, thoughts, and emotions consistently shape your reality in an effortless and fulfilling way.

Living by the principles of manifestation means you are constantly setting clear intentions, embodying gratitude and abundance, surrendering control, and trusting divine timing. Instead of reacting to life with frustration, fear, or doubt, you begin to see every experience - positive or challenging - as part of your path. You trust everything is unfolding exactly as it should, even if you cannot see the bigger picture. Over time, this trust strengthens, and manifestation becomes second nature rather than something you must consciously practice.

The key to making manifestation a way of life is aligning your thoughts, emotions, and actions with the reality you want to experience. It means embodying the person you aspire to be now and not waiting for external circumstances to change.

" It is about choosing abundance over lack, love over fear, and faith over doubt in every situation."

Teanna

The more you practice this, the easier it becomes, and soon, you will notice that the things you once struggled to manifest come to you effortlessly.

By adopting manifestation as a lifestyle, you move in harmony with the seasons of life, embracing cycles of growth, refinement, and transformation. You understand that everything happens in divine timing and that your role is not to control but to flow, trust, and take inspired action when the moment is right. When manifestation becomes a way of life, you no longer wish for things - you live as if they are already yours. The Cosmos responds by aligning your external reality with your inner state.

Becoming aligned with the Cosmic flow requires time, persistence, and daily practice, like refining your senses of taste, smell, and hearing or learning to cook or play the piano. You can experience daily peace, purpose, and fulfilment by embracing the flow. This approach enables you to navigate challenges with a broader perspective, fully embrace joy, and cultivate deeper connections with yourself and others.

Here are some practical ways to incorporate this belief into your everyday living:

Practice Presence
'Being In The Now' and Mindfulness

One of the best ways to embrace this mindset is to engage with the present moment fully. Since our human experience is temporary, every moment is an opportunity to feel, observe, and appreciate life truly. Practising mindfulness - whether through deep breathing, meditation, object observation, or simply paying attention to daily activities, i.e. in the shower, tea making, walking or eating - can help ground us in the now. Instead of rushing through life, please slow down and experience it fully. When you focus on the moment you are in, you stop worrying about the past or the future.

> **TRY** Start with simple mindfulness practices like object observation, deep breathing, body scans, or mindful walking to help you connect to the present moment. Over time, this will build an awareness that enables you to notice signs and synchronicities guiding you. You will see that life consists of magical moments that often seem too perfect to be coincidences.

This is the Cosmic Flow's way of guiding you, so stay open to synchronicities, signs, and unexpected opportunities. Pay attention to repeating patterns, numbers, or coincidences that feel significant. Trust these as cues pointing you in the right direction, especially when you think life is busy, chaotic, or stressful. These signs tell you to "Trust and Flow" and that everything happens for a reason.

> **TRY** Use 'Scan' throughout the day. Pause and be STILL. Take a few deep breaths and be CHILL. Then, be AWARE and notice your surroundings, how your body feels, and what emotions arise. This simple act brings awareness to the present moment. Then, you can move on to the NOW with more awareness.

Re-frame Challenges as Lessons

If we are spiritual beings here to grow, then every challenge is an opportunity for expansion. Instead of seeing difficulties as punishments or failures, shift your perspective to ask, "What can I learn from this?" or "Why is this happening FOR me?" Life's hardships often shape our strength, wisdom, and resilience.

This is something I know well. "Working through over a decade of chronic pain - had to be worth something, right?" And just that question set me on a path to change "what happened to me" and re-frame it to "why did it happen FOR me?" If I had not gone through what I did, I would not be here now writing this; I would not have seen my children every single day, eaten dinner with them around a table most nights, I would not appreciate the small things in life, the smell of a rose wafting through the window, the sight of a rainbow in the sky, the dance of a butterfly - all of which leave me in awe. I would not have spent years researching neurology or psychology. I would not have been in a position to save three people from suicide or help another into hospital during a Bipolar mania episode, having the skill set to stay with her and keep her calm for over 26 hours. I would not have opened up and accepted my spiritual gifts and met the most amazing people worldwide, bringing peace to many. I would not have held space for over 14000 people and found my path to meditation - my calling - my soul's purpose.

So, the next time you face a problem, instead of reacting with frustration, take a moment to reflect. This approach transforms obstacles into valuable life lessons.

- What is this teaching me?
- How can I grow from this?
- What perspective can I shift?

Let Go of Material Attachments

While material possessions can bring comfort, they are not the source of true happiness. If we view life as a temporary experience, we realise that status, wealth, and external validation are fleeting. What matters most is the love we give, the connections we create, and the wisdom we gain.

 I would like you to reflect on what truly brings you fulfilment. Is it possessions, experiences, relationships, and moments of joy? Practice gratitude for the intangibles in life - like kindness, love, and personal growth.

 Approach Life with Curiosity and Playfulness

If we are here to experience life, why not embrace it with curiosity and joy? Instead of fearing the unknown, approach new situations with wonder. Try new things, explore different perspectives, and allow yourself to play, create, and enjoy without the pressure of perfection.

 Do something new this week - try a new hobby, visit a place you have never been, or engage in a spontaneous activity. Even sitting in a different chair in your lounge or around the dining table changes your perspective! Approach it with childlike curiosity, without overthinking or self-judgment.

Cultivate Love and Compassion

Recognising that everyone is on their soul journey can make us more compassionate. People are doing the best they can with their current level of awareness and experiences. Instead of judging others, try to see them as fellow souls navigating their human experiences.

Follow Your Joy and Passions

You are aligned with your soul's purpose when you do what makes you happy. Your passions are a direct link to the Cosmic Flow. Therefore, pay attention to the activities or people that make you feel truly alive. These often point to the direction you are meant to be headed. Whether it is a hobby, a project, or simply spending time with loved ones. Following joy aligns you with the flow (See page 94) for finding your soul's purpose)

Embrace Gratitude Daily

Since life is temporary, cherish every moment. Gratitude shifts our focus from what is missing to what we have. It reminds us that even the simplest things - a smile, fresh air, a kind word - are profound gifts. By focusing on what you are grateful for, you attract more of what you want into your life. Start a gratitude journal, create a gratitude jar, or take a moment to appreciate the little things each day. This practice helps shift your energy, making you more receptive to abundance and positive experiences.

> **TRY** Every morning or night, list three things that you are grateful for. This practice trains your mind to focus on the beauty of life, no matter what challenges arise. Living with the understanding that we are spirit, having a human experience allows us to approach life with more purpose, love, and awareness. It encourages us to be present, embrace challenges as growth opportunities, connect with our inner selves, and live with greater freedom and joy.

The next time someone upsets you, pause before reacting. Ask yourself: What might they be going through? How can I respond with kindness? Shifting to a heart-centered approach fosters more profound, more meaningful connections.

Trust the Flow of Life - Surrender and Let Go of Resistance

Cosmic flow means embracing life's natural ebb and flow, including its challenges and changes. Instead of resisting, approach change with curiosity and openness. View challenges as opportunities for growth and learn to let go of expectations and attachments, knowing that everything happens as it is meant to.

Embrace life unfolding, even if it does not look exactly as planned. Trust that a more significant force is guiding you. When we view life as a temporary experience, we realise we do not need to control everything. Life unfolds as it is meant to, and trusting this process can bring immense peace. So, instead of resisting change, allow yourself to flow with it.

Trust in Divine Timing

Patience is an essential aspect of the Cosmic Flow. Sometimes, things do not happen when we want them to, but that does not mean they will not occur at the right time. Trust the timing, and things will unfold when you are truly ready for them, so let go of rushing and allow things to develop in their own time. When faced with uncertainty, remind yourself: "I am here to experience, learn, and grow. Everything is happening for my highest good." Trusting life unfolding can reduce anxiety and create a greater sense of ease.

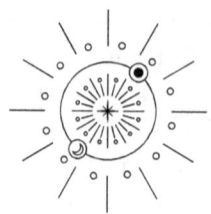

"Become one with cosmic energy and flow with it"

— Teanna

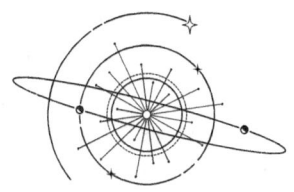

Feeling Cosmic Energy

"When you align with natural rhythms, you open yourself to a life of abundance and fulfilment."

Teanna

To align with Cosmic Energy, we have to feel it, and we do this via our energetic field, often called an aura or, in scientific terms, a biofield. This electromagnetic field of energy surrounds all of us and is measured in frequencies (Hertz Hz).

Ever wonder why you do not like someone when they walk up to you, yet you have not met them yet? That is your electromagnetic field (aura/biofield) at work - your energy has already been exchanged as you walk up to each other, and your intuition tells you something is off with its energetic frequency.

Everything in the Cosmos - from the cells in your body to the stars in the sky - is governed by frequencies. These vibrations influence brain function, physical health, emotions and consciousness. While some frequencies, like EMFs, stress-induced sound waves, and artificial light, can be disruptive, others, such as natural Earth frequencies, sound healing, and biological rhythms, can enhance mental clarity, emotional balance, and physical well-being. Understanding and working with these frequencies can lead to a healthier, more harmonious life where both mind and body function optimally.

Many people start their energy awareness journey as children, but it is never nurtured like our other senses. However, many are born naturally more aware of energy frequency reading, highly intuitive, empathetic, healing others, or contacting past loved ones. It is an ability we all have, but it gets confusing because it is not nurtured. So many, like myself, block it, and some sit silently with the awareness for years.

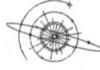 ## This is not woo-woo; this is science

Many kinds of energy frequencies can now be recorded in the human body. For instance, the heart's electrical activity can be recorded via ECG, and the brain's electrical activity can be measured with EEG. Cells also emit low levels of light (biophotons), and neurons create electrical impulses that produce detectable magnetic fields. However, scientists currently lack the tools to detect the subtle energies within the body on which practitioners like energy healers base their work.

But that does not mean they are not there or that humans cannot detect them. I have explained at a quantum level that everything vibrates energy, and frequencies play a fundamental role in shaping reality. String theory suggests that the smallest building blocks of matter are vibrating strings of energy and zero-point energy, the lowest possible energy state of quantum fields, which exist everywhere in space. It is there at the tiniest possible speck, and humans can feel and manipulate it with practice and awareness.

Then we have 'Earth Energy', which emits a fundamental electromagnetic frequency called the Schumann Resonance (7.83 Hz), which is believed to influence human brainwaves, mental clarity, and overall well-being. Studies suggest that when humans are exposed to this natural frequency, they experience improved focus, relaxation, and stress reduction. Conversely, disconnection from the Earth's natural field - such as prolonged exposure to artificial EMFs - can disrupt sleep cycles, immune function and cognitive balance. As I have explained, Cosmic frequencies, such as those emitted by planetary movements, influence human mood, energy levels, and even internal rhythms. Some research suggests solar flares and geomagnetic storms can impact melatonin production, leading to sleep disturbances and mood fluctuations.

We can also now record electromagnetic frequencies (EMFs), electric and magnetic energy waves that travel through space and affect technology and biological systems. These include radio waves, microwaves, infrared and visible light, ultraviolet (UV) rays, X-rays and gamma rays.

Understanding these and measuring them is important as not all energy frequencies are safe, such as lower frequency waves, i.e., radio and microwaves. Also, higher frequency waves, such as X-rays and gamma rays, are harmful, causing DNA damage and increasing cancer risk. EMFs also influence the brain and body - excessive exposure to artificial EMFs (from WiFi, mobile phones, and electronics) have been linked to sleep disturbances, headaches and oxidative stress. However, exposure to natural EMFs, such as the Earth's electromagnetic field (Schumann Resonance), may help regulate circadian rhythms and brain function.

We can also measure 'sound frequencies,' which are vibrational energy that travels as mechanical waves and directly impact brain function, emotions, and physical health. Different sound frequencies like Solfeggio and Binaural Beats can calm or stimulate the nervous system. Low frequencies (e.g., 40 Hz) are linked to deep relaxation, while high frequencies (e.g., 528 Hz, known as the "love frequency") may promote DNA repair and emotional healing. Studies suggest that music therapy and exposure to healing sound vibrations can reduce stress, anxiety and even pain perception by stimulating dopamine and serotonin production in the brain. In contrast, prolonged exposure to chaotic or dissonant noise can increase cortisol levels, leading to stress and mental fatigue.

I get a lot of feedback from my meditation groups about how they seem to go deeper and get more from my meditations than others. I usually facilitate three types of meditations back to back: mindfulness, body relaxation, and guided. I thought it was down to my method.

But I also get a lot of compliments on my voice, so I had its frequency analysed and was very humbled at the results. My voice naturally resonates at 144Hz!, which is known to link to a lot of the Cosmic energy frequencies. I have listed these in the cut out, as you will see I was blown away.

144 Hz

" Your voice's natural frequency at 144 Hz suggests a resonance with balance, healing, and universal harmony. It carries a calming, harmonising energy that is powerful in meditation, healing practices, or communication. enhancing clarity, emotional well-being, and connection to the Cosmos."

144 Hz enhances harmony with nature and promotes healing, linked to the Earth's Schumann Resonance (7.83 Hz) and its harmonics. It acts as a grounding frequency, significant in balance and connection. In healing practices, 144 Hz is a "manifestation" frequency associated with DNA repair, higher consciousness, and mental clarity. It is also connected to the Fibonacci Sequence and the Golden Ratio, reflecting natural growth and universal harmony. Also linked to the Heart Chakra, it promotes love and healing, and is associated with the activation of the Third Eye and Crown Chakras. In spiritual texts, the number 144 holds significance, seen as the frequency of "divine light" or "Cosmic awakening."

Science is at a stage where it has the tools to measure all the frequencies listed in Hz but does not yet have the technology to measure the more subtle frequencies, such as spiritual and metaphysical vibrations, which influence human consciousness, emotional states, and manifestation abilities. But in time, I believe these will be recordable.

Before such a time, you must learn to feel the Cosmic Energy in your aura and use your intuition to decipher it. Intuition is your inner compass; we are all born with it but are not taught to nurture it. Cosmic Flow invites you to trust this guidance rather than overthinking or seeking constant approval from others. Practice listening to your gut feelings and acting based on your inner wisdom. Over time, you will notice that your intuition becomes clearer and more reliable as you move further into the flow - listen to energy awareness exercises online.

Since we are more than just our bodies and minds, it is important to nurture our spiritual sides. This could mean journaling, meditation, affirmations, or simply spending time in nature. The goal is to connect with the deeper part of you that exists beyond daily stress and responsibilities. This is where manifestation is also felt, and you become more aware of synchronisations around you. By integrating these practices into your life, you can feel more in tune with the Cosmic Flow and experience greater peace, clarity, and purpose.

A meditation practice is a must, as it is one of the most powerful tools for tuning into the flow of the Cosmos. Through meditation, you can quiet the mind and create space to listen to your inner guidance. This can help you align with the natural rhythm of life, feel more at peace, and understand your true path. If you only meditate for a few minutes each morning or evening, you will begin a practice of growth. My meditations can be found online.

Take 5 - 10 minutes a day for stillness. Close your eyes, focus on your breath, and listen to your inner self. Ask, "What do I need today?" This simple check-in fosters inner peace and clarity.

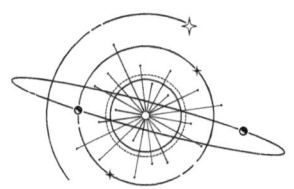

Overcoming Challenges
Limiting Beliefs and Self Sabotage

On the manifestation journey, you can encounter several challenges. The most common self-inflicted ones are 'Limiting Beliefs' and 'Self-Sabotage'.

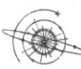**Limiting Beliefs**

They are like self-imposed shackles that hinder progress and diminish potential, often rooted in early experiences. They manifest as negative self-talk, reinforcing feelings of inadequacy and preventing individuals from stepping outside their comfort zones. Research shows that individuals create a foundation for resilience and success by questioning and replacing these beliefs with empowering ones.

Ultimately, overcoming these beliefs is about achieving success, realising your inherent potential, and leading a more fulfilling life.

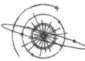**Self Sabotage**

This is deliberately or unconsciously hindering your progress, success, or well-being. It often stems from deep-seated fears, limiting beliefs, or unresolved emotional patterns that lead individuals to engage in behaviours that undermine their goals. This can manifest in various ways, such as procrastination, negative self-talk, perfectionism, self-doubt, or unhealthy habits that contradict personal or professional aspirations.

Psychologists suggest that self-sabotage is often driven by fear of failure, fear of success, or low self-worth, making individuals subconsciously create obstacles.

For example, someone striving for career growth might consistently miss deadlines or avoid opportunities due to a fear of not being good enough. Similarly, individuals may push people away in relationships to protect themselves from potential hurt.

Overcoming self-sabotage requires self-awareness, identifying negative thought patterns, and actively challenging behaviours that hinder progress.

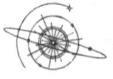

Techniques

Cognitive-behavioural therapy (CBT), mindfulness, and self-compassion can help break these cycles, allowing individuals to build healthier habits and work toward their true potential.

You can also overcome these by converting a Limiting Belief into an Empowered belief and then into a personal Affirmation to which you attach a positive emotion.

 Steps to Internalise Empowering Beliefs

Acknowledge the Limiting Beliefs
On the following pages, circle all the ' limiting beliefs' that resonate with you.

Change to Empowering Beliefs
Find the counter-empowering beliefs page 168

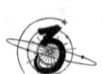
Now Turn them into Affirmations
Examples can be found on page 172

Remember to write it in the first person, present tense, and make it specific. For example: "I embrace my worth and know I am enough in every situation."

The more you say or write an affirmation - with emotion - the more your subconscious absorbs it. Aim for at least 2 - 3 times a day. See page 108 how to work with these affirmations.

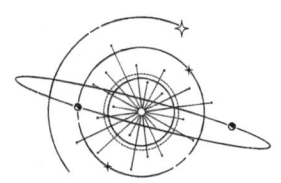

Limiting Beliefs

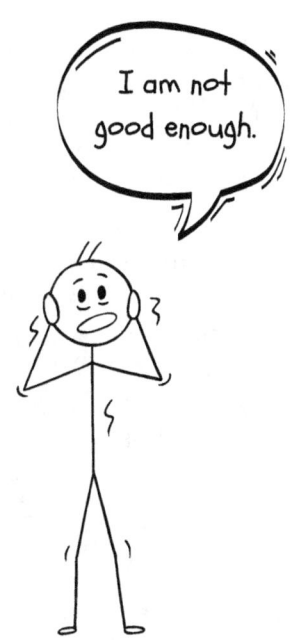

Limiting Beliefs

Self - Worth and Personal Growth
1. I am not good enough.
2. I do not deserve success or happiness.
3. I cannot change who I am.
4. People will judge me if I fail.
5. I am too old to start something new.
6. I am too young to be taken seriously.
7. I need to be perfect to be loved.
8. Mistakes define me.
9. I cannot trust myself to make good decisions.
10. I will never be as good as others.

Relationships
11. I am unlovable.
12. All relationships end in heartbreak.
13. People always leave me.
14. Love requires sacrifice and suffering.
15. I cannot be happy without a partner.
16. People only like me for what I can do for them.
17. Vulnerability leads to rejection.
18. I do not deserve healthy relationships.
19. I have to fix others to be valuable.
20. Conflict means the relationship is failing.

Money and Abundance
21. Money is the root of all evil.
22. Rich people are greedy or selfish.
23. I am not smart enough to manage money.
24. I will never make enough money.
25. I cannot afford to follow my dreams.
26. Financial success is only for lucky people.
27. Saving money means missing out on life.
28. I do not deserve wealth.
29. It is selfish to want more money.
30. There is never enough to go around

Career and Success
31. Success requires sacrificing happiness.
32. I am not talented enough to succeed.
33. Failure means I am not capable.
34. Networking feels fake and manipulative.
35. I cannot start a business without a lot of money.
36. I am not a leader.
37. My dreams are unrealistic.
38. It is too late to change my career.
39. I do not have the time to pursue my goals.
40. Success is only for certain types of people.

Health and Wellness
41. I will always struggle with my weight.
42. Healthy living is too hard.
43. My genetics determine my health.
44. I am too busy to take care of myself.

Limiting Beliefs

45. I am not disciplined enough to stick to a routine.
46. Exercise is a punishment, not a reward.
47. Eating healthy is expensive.
48. I cannot recover from my past health issues.
49. I will never feel confident in my body.
50. Pain is something I have to live with.

Time
51. There is never enough time.
52. I am always behind everyone else.
53. I need to hustle constantly to get ahead.
54. I cannot take breaks without falling behind.
55. I have to do everything myself.
56. If I relax, I am being lazy.
57. I cannot manage my time well.
58. Life is a race against the clock.
59. Time works against me.
60. My dreams take too long to achieve.

Creativity
61. I am not a creative person.
62. Nobody wants to hear what I have to say.
63. My ideas aren't original enough.
64. Creative work does not pay the bills.
65. I do not have the talent to succeed in art.
66. Sharing my work makes me vulnerable to criticism.
67. I need to follow trends to be successful.
68. Creativity is a waste of time.
69. I cannot learn new skills as an adult.
70. It is too late to pursue my artistic passions.

Spirituality and Purpose
71. Life is meaningless.
72. I am disconnected from my higher self.
73. I do not have a purpose in life.
74. I am not worthy of divine love or guidance.
75. I cannot trust the Cosmos to support me.
76. Meditation or spiritual practices do not work for me.
77. Enlightenment is only for spiritual gurus.
78. My past mistakes make me spiritually unworthy.
79. I am not intuitive enough to understand my path.
80. Spiritual growth is too difficult or time - consuming.

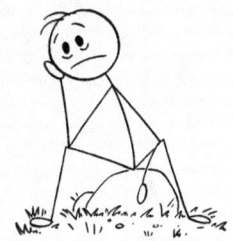

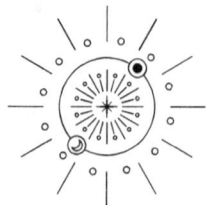

"Challenges are what make life interesting, and overcoming them is what makes life meaningful"

Joshua J. Marine

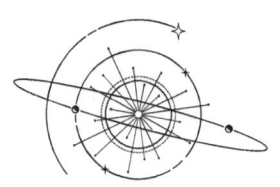

Empowering Beliefs

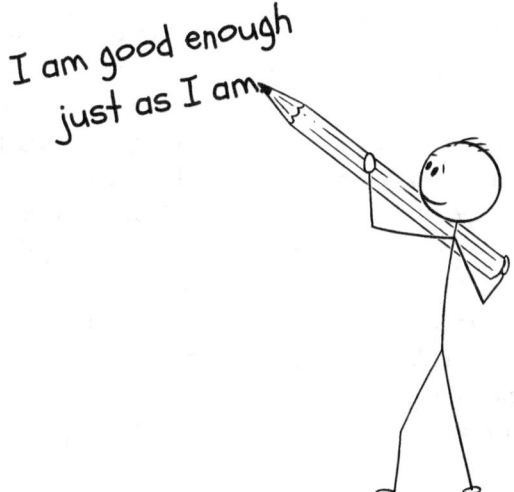

Empowering Beliefs

Self Worth
1. I am good enough just as I am.
2. I deserve success and happiness.
3. I have the power to change and grow.
4. Failure is a stepping stone to success, not a judgment of my worth.
5. it is never too late to start something new.
6. My age is an asset; I bring value and perspective.
7. I am loved for being my authentic self, not for being perfect.
8. Mistakes are opportunities to learn and grow.
9. I trust myself to make decisions that align with my values.
10. My unique path makes me incomparable to others.

Relationships
11. I am deeply lovable and worthy of love.
12. Every relationship is an opportunity for growth and connection.
13. I am surrounded by people who value and appreciate me.
14. Love is a source of joy, not sacrifice or suffering.
15. I am whole and complete on my own; love enhances my life.
16. People value me for who I am, not just what I do for them.
17. Vulnerability creates deeper, meaningful connections.
18. I deserve and cultivate healthy, fulfilling relationships.
19. I do not need to fix others to feel valuable; my presence is enough.
20. Conflict is an opportunity to communicate and grow, not a sign of failure.

Money and Abundance
21. Money is a tool that can be used for good and positive change.
22. Wealthy people can be kind, generous, and ethical.
23. I am capable of managing my money with confidence and ease.
24. I have the skills and determination to create financial abundance.
25. My dreams are worth investing in, and the Cosmos supports me.
26. I create my own luck through hard work and belief in myself.
27. Saving money allows me to create the life I want without missing out.
28. I deserve to be financially secure and abundant.
29. Wanting more money is a reflection of my desire to grow and share.
30. There is enough abundance in the world for everyone, including me.

Empowering Beliefs

Career and Success

31. Success is a journey I can enjoy while staying true to myself.
32. My unique talents and efforts pave the way for my success.
33. Failure is an important part of my growth and development.
34. Building genuine relationships is a key part of networking.
35. I can start a business with creativity, passion, and resourcefulness.
36. I am a leader in my own right, with my unique style and strengths.
37. My dreams are achievable, and I take steps toward them every day.
38. It is never too late to pursue a career that aligns with my passions.
39. I prioritise my goals and make time for what matters most.
40. Success is available to everyone, including me.

Health and Wellness

41. I can cultivate a healthy body and mind with compassion and patience.
42. Healthy living is enjoyable and enriching.
43. I can make choices that positively impact my health, regardless of genetics.
44. Taking care of myself is a priority, not an inconvenience.
45. I have the discipline to create routines that support my wellness.
46. Exercise is a gift to my body and mind, not a punishment.
47. Eating healthy is an investment in myself and my future.
48. My body has incredible healing potential, and I honour it.
49. I can love and respect my body at every stage of its journey.
50. I can take steps to improve my physical and emotional comfort.

Time

51. I have all the time I need to do what is most important.
52. I am exactly where I am meant to be at this moment.
53. Resting and recharging makes me more productive and fulfilled.
54. Taking breaks allows me to approach tasks with renewed energy.
55. Delegating tasks helps me accomplish more with ease.
56. Resting is a form of self - care, not laziness.
57. I manage my time effectively and honour my priorities.
58. Life unfolds at the perfect pace for me.
59. Time is a tool I can use to create the life I want.
60. Small, consistent steps lead me to achieve my dreams.

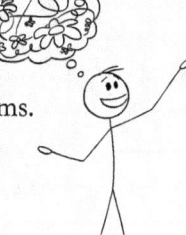

Empowering Beliefs

Creativity and Expression

61. I am creative in my own unique way.
62. My voice and perspective matter and are worth sharing.
63. My ideas are valuable and have the power to inspire others.
64. Creativity can bring joy and abundance into my life.
65. My talent grows with practice, patience, and dedication.
66. Sharing my work connects me to others and builds resilience.
67. I succeed by staying true to my authentic self, not by following trends.
68. Creativity enriches my life and is never a waste of time.
69. I can learn new skills and grow creatively at any age.
70. My artistic passions are worth pursuing at any stage of life.

Spirituality and Purpose

71. Life has profound meaning, and I can create purpose in every moment.
72. I am deeply connected to my higher self and the Cosmos.
73. I have a unique purpose that contributes to the greater good.
74. I am worthy of divine love and guidance simply because I exist.
75. The Cosmos supports me and provides for my highest good.
76. Meditation and spiritual practices align me with peace and clarity.
77. Spiritual growth is accessible to anyone willing to seek it.
78. My past mistakes are lessons that deepen my spiritual journey.
79. I trust my intuition to guide me toward my highest path.
80. Spiritual growth is a joyful process of discovery and connection.

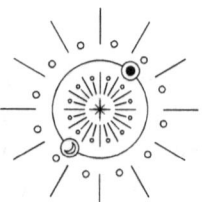

"Whatever you hold in your mind on a consistent basis is exactly what you will experience in your life."

Tony Robbins

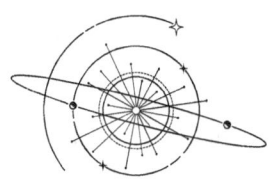

Personal Affirmations

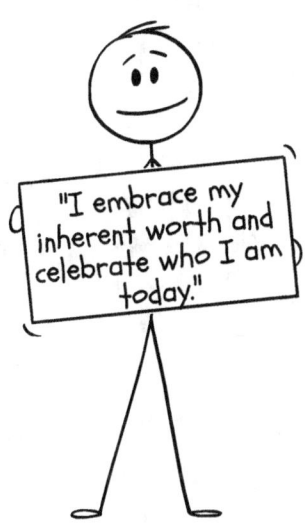

Affirmations are positive statements or intentions repeated to reprogram the mind, shift perspectives, or manifest desired changes. They work by influencing thought patterns and emotional states. This approach is thought to harmonise mental and physical states by aligning our internal dialogue with our energetic qualities.

Affirmations should be personal to you and either written, said or sung with attached emotions.

Creating personal affirmations can be tricky when you first start writing personal affirmations, so here are some sample affirmations for each limiting belief section. Use these as your base affirmations, and change them to make them personal.

On my website - www.TeannaTaylor.com - you will find some affirmations to print out and others set to music. See page 114 about working with affirmations.

Money flows with ease and grace,
Abundance fills my scared space.
Opportunities me, both big and small.
Wealth and joy, I claim it all!

Love flows to me, strong and true,
a bond so deep, forever new.
With open heart, I call my pair.
a love so kind, beyond compare.

My body heals, my spirit glows,
with every breath, my energy flows.
Strength and health are here to stay,
I feel more vibrant every day!

Empowering Beliefs About Self-Worth and Personal Growth

1. I am good enough, just as I am.
Affirmation: "I embrace my inherent worth and celebrate who I am today."

2. I deserve success and happiness.
Affirmation: "I open my heart to the success and happiness that is my birthright."

3. I have the power to change and grow.
Affirmation: "I trust in my ability to evolve and create the life I desire."

4. Failure is a stepping stone to success, not a judgment of my worth.
Affirmation: "Each setback is a powerful opportunity for me to grow stronger and wiser."

5. It is never too late to start something new.
Affirmation: "Every day brings a fresh start, and I confidently embrace new beginnings."

6. My age is an asset; I bring value and perspective.
Affirmation: "My experiences enrich my journey and empower my unique contributions."

7. I am loved for being my authentic self, not for being perfect.
Affirmation: "I am deeply loved and accepted just as I am."

8. Mistakes are opportunities to learn and grow.
Affirmation: "I learn and thrive from every experience, and mistakes guide me toward wisdom."

9. I trust myself to make decisions that align with my values.
Affirmation: "I honour my inner wisdom and trust it to guide my choices."

10. My unique path makes me incomparable to others.
Affirmation: "I walk my path with confidence and pride, knowing it is uniquely mine."

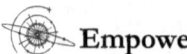 **Empowering Beliefs About Relationships**

1. I am profoundly lovable and worthy of love.
Affirmation: "I radiate love and attract meaningful, loving connections."

2. Every relationship is an opportunity for growth and connection.
Affirmation: "I welcome growth and deeper understanding through my relationships."

3. I am surrounded by people who value and appreciate me.
Affirmation: "I am deeply cherished by those who see and honour my worth."

4. Love is a source of joy, not sacrifice or suffering.
Affirmation: "Love brings harmony and joy into my life."

5. I am whole and completely independent; love enhances my life.
Affirmation: "I am whole and embrace love as a beautiful addition to my journey."

6. People value me for who I am, not just what I do for them.
Affirmation: "I am valued for my essence, not my actions."

7. Vulnerability creates deeper, meaningful connections.
Affirmation: "My openness strengthens the bonds I share with others."

8. I deserve and cultivate healthy, fulfilling relationships.
Affirmation: "I nurture relationships that align with my highest good."

9. I do not need to fix others to feel valuable; my presence is enough.
Affirmation: "My being is enough to make a positive difference in the lives of others."

10. Conflict is an opportunity to communicate and grow, not a sign of failure.
Affirmation: "Through open communication, conflict leads to greater understanding and connection."

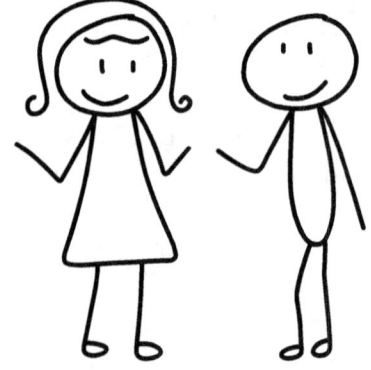

Empowering Beliefs About Money and Abundance

1. Money is a tool that can be used for good and positive change.
Affirmation: "I use money as a tool to create abundance and contribute to the greater good."

2. Wealthy people can be kind, generous, and ethical.
Affirmation: "I align wealth with kindness, generosity, and integrity."

3. I am capable of managing my money with confidence and ease.
Affirmation: "I handle my finances with wisdom and confidence."

4. I have the skills and determination to create financial abundance.
Affirmation: "My skills and determination attract financial success with ease."

5. My dreams are worth investing in, and the Cosmos supports me.
Affirmation: "I invest in my dreams, knowing the Cosmos supports my vision."

6. I create my own luck through hard work and belief in myself.
Affirmation: "I manifest opportunities through my actions and unwavering belief in myself."

7. Saving money allows me to create the life I want without missing out.
Affirmation: "I save intentionally, creating a future full of possibilities."

8. I deserve to be financially secure and abundant.
Affirmation: "Financial security and abundance flow freely to me."

9. Wanting more money is a reflection of my desire to grow and share.
Affirmation: "My desire for wealth reflects my purpose to grow and give generously."

10. There is enough abundance in the world for everyone, including me.
Affirmation: "The world's abundance flows to me and others with ease and grace."

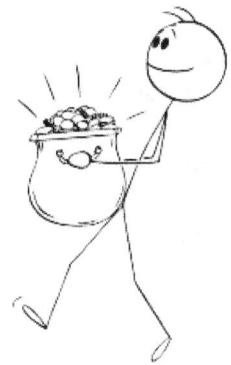

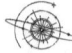 **Empowering Beliefs About Career and Success**

1. Success is a journey I can enjoy while staying true to myself. Affirmation: "I enjoy every step of my journey, honouring my authentic self as I succeed."

2. My unique talents and efforts pave the way for my success.
Affirmation: "I trust my unique talents to guide me toward meaningful success."

3. Failure is an important part of my growth and development.
Affirmation: "Every failure brings valuable lessons that strengthen my growth."

4. Building genuine relationships is a key part of networking.
Affirmation: "I create authentic connections that enrich my personal and professional life."

5. I can start a business with creativity, passion, and resourcefulness.
Affirmation: "My creativity and determination empower me to build a thriving business."

6. I am a leader in my own right, with my unique style and strengths.
Affirmation: "I lead with confidence, authenticity, and purpose."

7. My dreams are achievable, and I take steps toward them every day.
Affirmation: "I turn my dreams into reality through consistent and inspired action."

8. Pursuing a career that aligns with my passions is never too late.
Affirmation: "I am never too late to follow my passions and create a fulfilling career."

9. I prioritise my goals and make time for what matters most.
Affirmation: "I focus on my priorities and devote my energy to what truly matters."

10. Success is available to everyone, including me.
Affirmation: "Success is abundant, and I claim my share with gratitude and joy."

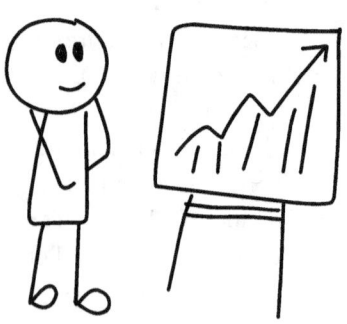

Empowering Beliefs About Health and Wellness

1. I can cultivate a healthy body and mind with compassion and patience.
Affirmation: "I nurture my body and mind with love, patience, and care."

2. Healthy living is enjoyable and enriching.
Affirmation: "I embrace healthy choices as a source of joy and fulfilment."

3. I can make choices that positively impact my health, regardless of genetics.
Affirmation: "I am empowered to make choices that uplift my health and vitality."

4. Taking care of myself is a priority, not an inconvenience.
Affirmation: "I honour my well-being by prioritising self-care every day."

5. I have the discipline to create routines that support my wellness.
Affirmation: "I establish and enjoy routines that nurture my body, mind, and spirit."

6. Exercise is a gift to my body and mind, not a punishment.
Affirmation: "I move my body with joy and gratitude for its strength and resilience."

7. Eating healthy is an investment in myself and my future.
Affirmation: "I nourish my body with food that supports my energy and well-being."

8. My body has incredible healing potential, and I honour it.
Affirmation: "I trust in my body's innate ability to heal and thrive."

9. I can love and respect my body at every stage of its journey.
Affirmation: "I celebrate and honour my body at every stage of its transformation."

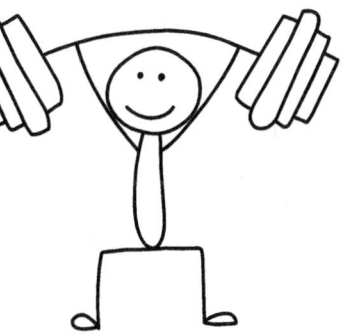

10. I can take steps to improve my physical and emotional comfort.
Affirmation: "I take mindful steps every day to enhance my health and emotional balance."

Empowering Beliefs About Time

1. I have all the time I need to do what is most important.
Affirmation: "I focus on what matters most, trusting time to work in my favour."

2. I am exactly where I am meant to be at this moment.
Affirmation: "I embrace the present moment, knowing it is perfect for my growth."

3. Resting and recharging makes me more productive and fulfilled.
Affirmation: "Rest fuels my energy and brings clarity to my purpose."

4. Taking breaks allows me to approach tasks with renewed energy.
Affirmation: "I step away when needed, trusting that I will return with fresh energy."

5. Delegating tasks helps me accomplish more with ease.
Affirmation: "I trust others and share responsibilities to achieve greater harmony."

6. Resting is a form of self - care, not laziness. Affirmation: "I honour my needs by allowing myself time to rest and recharge."

7. I manage my time effectively and honour my priorities.
Affirmation: "I focus my time and energy on what truly matters to me."

8. Life unfolds at the perfect pace for me.
Affirmation: "I trust the flow of my life and embrace its perfect timing."

9. Time is a tool I can use to create the life I want.
Affirmation: "I use time wisely and intentionally to build the life I envision."

10. Small, consistent steps lead me to achieve my dreams.
Affirmation: "I make steady progress toward my goals with patience and determination."

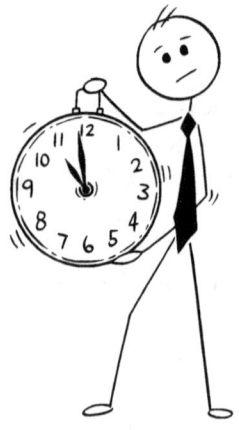

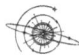 **Empowering Beliefs About Creativity and Expression**

1. I am creative in my own unique way.
Affirmation: "My creativity flows freely and authentically in all that I do."

2. My voice and perspective matter and are worth sharing.
Affirmation: "My voice is powerful, and my perspective enriches the world."

3. My ideas are valuable and have the power to inspire others.
Affirmation: "My ideas inspire change and create meaningful connections."

4. Creativity can bring joy and abundance into my life.
Affirmation: "I welcome creativity as a joyful and abundant force in my life."

5. My talent grows with practice, patience, and dedication.
Affirmation: "I nurture my talents, knowing they grow with practice and care."

6. Sharing my work connects me to others and builds resilience.
Affirmation: "I share my creations with confidence, knowing they foster connection."

7. I succeed by staying true to my authentic self, not by following trends.
Affirmation: "My authenticity shines through in all that I create and share."

8. Creativity enriches my life and is never a waste of time.
Affirmation: "Creativity is a sacred and meaningful part of my life's journey."

9. I can learn new skills and grow creatively at any age.
Affirmation: "I embrace learning as a constant, joyful part of my creative journey."

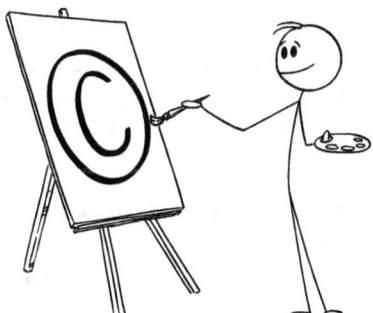

10. My artistic passions are worth pursuing at any stage of life.
Affirmation: "My passions enrich my life and deserve my time and energy at any stage."

Empowering Beliefs About Spirituality and Purpose

1. Life has profound meaning, and I can create purpose in every moment.
Affirmation: "I infuse meaning and purpose into every action I take."

2. I am deeply connected to my higher self and the Cosmos.
Affirmation: "I am in harmony with my higher self and the infinite wisdom of the Cosmos."

3. I have a unique purpose that contributes to the greater good.
Affirmation: "My purpose is a meaningful gift that serves the world."

4. I am worthy of divine love and guidance simply because I exist.
Affirmation: "I am deeply loved and guided by the divine in all that I do."

5. The Cosmos supports me and provides for my highest good.
Affirmation: "The Cosmos aligns everything for my highest good and greatest joy."

6. Meditation and spiritual practices align me with peace and clarity.
Affirmation: "Through meditation, I connect with peace, clarity, and divine wisdom."

7. Spiritual growth is accessible to anyone willing to seek it.
Affirmation: "I grow spiritually every day as I open my heart and mind to truth."

8. My past mistakes are lessons that deepen my spiritual journey.
Affirmation: "I honour my past as a sacred teacher that enriches my soul's path."

9. I trust my intuition to guide me toward my highest path.
Affirmation: "My intuition lights the way to my highest and truest self."

10. Spiritual growth is a joyful process of discovery and connection.
Affirmation: "I embrace spiritual growth as a joyful and infinite journey of love."

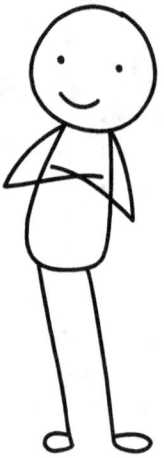

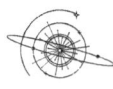
How to use your empowering beliefs and personal Affirmations

 Create a Daily Ritual
You can start your day by repeating the affirmation aloud or writing it down 3 - 5 times.

 Use visualisation
Imagine yourself living in alignment with the belief.

 Gratitude Integration
Pair your belief with gratitude. For example, "I am grateful for the unique qualities that make me enough."

 Track Small Wins
Journal how you acted in alignment with the belief throughout the day. And celebrate progress by acknowledging even small shifts in mindset or actions that reflect your new belief.

 Anchor it in Emotions
Feel the truth of the affirmation as you say it. Pair it with gratitude, joy, or excitement.

 Display Reminders
Write affirmations on sticky notes and place them where you will see them (e.g., mirrors, desks, on the fridge, by the kettle or phone screensavers).

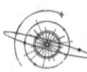
Other challenges you could face include:

 Lack of Clarity

Manifestation requires a clear vision of what you truly want. If your desires are vague or constantly changing, it becomes difficult to focus your energy and intentions effectively, and it confuses the RAS, which will not know clearly what to point out to you. Do the Ikigai and Life Balance Wheel to help you set meaningful, clear intentions.

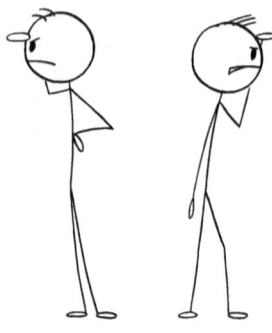

 Negative Energy and Emotional Blocks

Unresolved emotional wounds, past traumas, or lingering negative energy can block manifestations. Suppressed emotions such as guilt, resentment, or fear create resistance, preventing you from aligning with your goals.

To address these, the first step is to acknowledge and accept these emotions rather than ignoring or suppressing them. Journaling, meditation, and shadow work[5] are powerful tools for uncovering the root of these blocks and understanding their influence on your thoughts and actions.

Emotional energy must be processed and released to create space for positive manifestations. Practices such as breath work, energy cleansing, and forgiveness rituals help shift stagnant energy.

Re-framing limiting beliefs and replacing them with empowering affirmations can rewire your mindset, making it easier to attract what you desire. (see previous pages) Most importantly, self-compassion, deep inner healing and alignment.

 Impatience and Lack of Trust

Many people expect instant results, but manifestation is a process that unfolds at the right time and in the right way. When frustration and doubt creep in, they disrupt your energy flow, creating resistance that slows progress. The key is to shift from attachment to the outcome to a mindset of trust and allowing. Focus on small signs of progress, celebrate every step forward, and remind yourself that what you desire is already on its way.

---

(5) Shadow work is the process of exploring the unconscious parts of yourself - traits, emotions, and desires you may have rejected or hidden. It involves acknowledging and accepting these "shadow" aspects instead of ignoring or suppressing them. By doing shadow work, you can heal emotional wounds, break negative patterns, and grow into a more whole, authentic version of yourself.

Practices such as gratitude, mindfulness, and visualisation help reinforce belief in the process and keep your energy aligned with your intentions. Releasing control and surrendering to divine timing allows things to unfold effortlessly and in perfect alignment with your highest good. Instead of obsessing over when or how your manifestation will arrive, focus on becoming the person who is ready to receive it - because when the timing is right, everything will fall into place naturally.

 Fear of Change
Even when we desire something deeply, change can feel uncomfortable. The subconscious mind may resist new opportunities or success because it feels safer in familiar situations, even if they are unfulfilling.

This resistance is often rooted in past experiences, limiting beliefs, or fear of failure. The key is to reframe change as an opportunity for expansion rather than a risk. Instead of focusing on the fear of what could go wrong, shift your mindset to what could go right. Practices such as visualisation, affirmations, and small, intentional steps forward can help ease the transition. Trusting that the Cosmos is guiding you towards your highest good allows you to embrace change confidently rather than with resistance.

 External Influences and Doubt from Others
Surrounding yourself with sceptical or negative people can weaken your faith in manifestation. Constant criticism or discouragement from others can make you question your abilities or feel unworthy of your desires.

Strengthening your own belief in your manifestation journey is the first step to overcoming this. Protect your energy by setting boundaries with those who discourage you and choosing to engage with uplifting, supportive communities. Affirmations, journaling, and meditation can help reinforce your inner trust and keep you aligned with your goals despite external noise.

Instead of seeking validation from others, cultivate self-trust and inner knowing that what you desire is meant for you. Remember, your manifestation is your journey; not everyone will understand it, and that is okay.

Attachment to Outcomes

Obsessing over specific results and trying to control how things unfold can create resistance, so letting go and trusting the Cosmos is crucial. Manifestation works best when you focus on the feeling of having what you want rather than fixating on the exact path it must take. Overcoming this requires trust, surrender, and alignment with Cosmic flow. Instead of fixating on the exact path your desire must take, shift your focus to the feeling of already having it. Embrace faith and detachment, knowing that what is meant for you will come in the perfect way and timing. Practices like visualisation, gratitude, and affirmations can help reinforce this trust.

When you release control and remain open to limitless possibilities, you allow the Cosmos to work in your favour, often delivering something even greater than you imagined. Let go, trust the process, and flow with the unfolding of your manifestations.

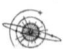 **Not Taking Action**

Manifestation is not just about visualisation and affirmations; it requires aligned action. Sitting back and waiting for things to happen without effort can delay or block manifestations. Inspired action is key.

Overcoming inaction in manifestation requires understanding that visualisation and affirmations alone are not enough - they must be paired with aligned, inspired action. Remember, the Cosmos responds to energy and movement, so simply waiting for things to happen without effort can create stagnation and delays.

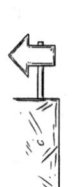
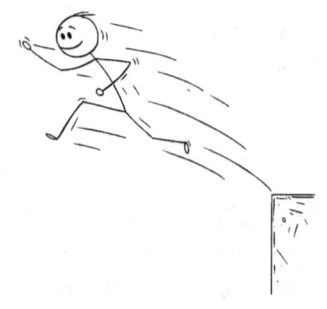

Taking small, intentional steps toward your goal signals to the Cosmos that you are ready to receive. Inspired action does not mean forcing things but rather following intuitive nudges, seizing opportunities, and staying open to synchronicities. Whether it is learning a new skill, reaching out to someone, or shifting your daily habits, each step brings you closer to your manifestation. Trust that the path will reveal itself as you move forward - because action creates momentum, and momentum brings manifestations to life.

Low Self - Worth

Feeling unworthy of success, love, or abundance can unconsciously push away opportunities. If you do not believe you deserve something deep down, you may unknowingly repel it.

Overcoming feelings of unworthiness is essential to allowing success, love, and abundance to flow into your life. If, deep down, you do not believe you deserve something, your subconscious mind may create self-sabotaging patterns that push opportunities away. To shift this, start by identifying and challenging limiting beliefs that tell you otherwise. Use affirmations, inner child healing[6] and self-love practices to reprogram your mind with the truth:

You are inherently worthy of everything you desire. Surround yourself with supportive, high-vibrational influences and practice gratitude for what you already have, reinforcing the energy of abundance. When you fully embrace your worth, you become an energetic match for your dreams, allowing success, love, and prosperity to flow to you effortlessly.

 Lack of Consistency

Manifestation requires consistency in thoughts, beliefs, and actions. If you frequently shift between faith and doubt, it sends mixed signals to the Cosmos and your RAS, making it harder to attract what you desire.

Overcoming this requires a commitment to your thoughts, beliefs, and actions. Manifestation thrives on energetic alignment and repetition; your thoughts, emotions, and actions must consistently match the reality you want to create. To stay aligned, develop a daily practice that reinforces your belief, such as affirmations, visualisation, journaling, and gratitude. Surround yourself with inspiring influences and regularly remind yourself why you started. Trust that the energy is building beneath the surface even if you do not see instant results.

 Burnout and Energy Drain

Constantly focusing on manifestation without balancing your energy can lead to burnout. If you are too fixated on the outcome, you may become exhausted and disconnected from the joy of the journey.

---

(6) Inner child healing is the practice of reconnecting with, understanding, and nurturing the younger version of yourself - especially the parts of you that experienced emotional pain, neglect, or unmet needs growing up.

Overcoming this requires balance, trust, and self-care. Manifestation is not about pushing or forcing but about aligning and allowing. If you feel drained, step back and focus on nourishing your energy through activities that bring you peace, such as meditation, time in nature, creative expression, or mindful movement. Trust that the Cosmos works behind the scenes even when you take a break. Shift your focus from the outcome to enjoying the present moment, reinforcing an energy of abundance and ease rather than stress. By balancing inspired action with rest, you stay energetically aligned and open to receiving your manifestations effortlessly.

Overview - How to Overcome These Challenges
- Practice self-awareness
- Recognise limiting patterns and address them
- Stay emotionally aligned
- Work on healing past traumas and releasing negativity
- Let go of control and embrace the flow of life
- Take inspired action
- Align your daily habits with your goals
- Surround yourself with positivity
- Seek supportive communities or mentors
- Detach from the outcome
- Believe that everything is working out for your highest good
- Trust the process

Addressing these challenges creates a clearer path for your manifestations to materialise and align with your highest potential.

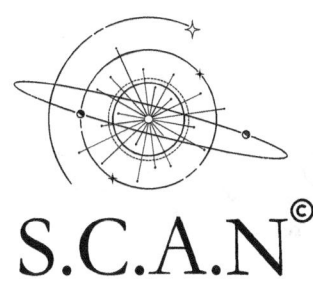

S.C.A.N©

S.C.A.N. is a new mindfulness practice that MJ and I formulated when writing our Rainbow Breath children's books. We received a lot of feedback from parents that it was working just as well for them! It can help whenever you are feeling overwhelmed or distressed.

You S.C.A.N., the inner you and the things which are going on around you. It allows for the creation of space to observe and tame your feelings. It helps you develop the emotional intelligence and the psychological flexibility required for greater mastery over challenging moments.

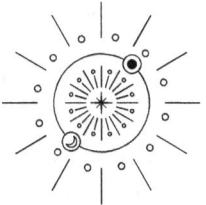

"Almost everything will work again if you unplug it for a few minutes, including you"

Anne Lamott

TRY S.C.A.N. is a new mindfulness practice that MJ and I formulated when writing our Rainbow Breath children's books. We received a lot of feedback from parents that it was working just as well for them! It can help whenever you are feeling overwhelmed or distressed.

You S.C.A.N. the inner you and the things which are going on around you. It allows for the creation of space to observe and tame your feelings. It helps you develop the emotional intelligence and the psychological flexibility required for greater mastery over challenging moments.

The four steps can take a few seconds to a few minutes to complete.

'S' stands for STILL

Be still, which means without moving, slow your breathing. This is a moment to pause, rest and breathe.

'C' stands for CHILL

It is time to chill and relax. Take a few deep, calm breaths, relax your muscles, and release any tension you feel in your body. Concentrate on breathing - feel the breath going in and out through your nose and expand your belly as you feel peace.

'A' stands for AWARE

Be aware of what has been happening inside and outside of you, including any thoughts, emotions, feelings, bodily sensations, sounds, sights - all the ongoing sensory input - without judging your experience.

Broaden your awareness to take in the circumstances. What caused you to feel overwhelmed or unbalanced? Notice how you can be in this situation without being ruled by it. Continue to breathe deeply.

'N' stands for NOW

Be in the now throughout your day. Use all of your senses to keep yourself mindful. Continue to observe your inner and outer experiences peacefully throughout your day.

If thoughts, feelings, and emotions begin to arise unbalanced or if your muscles tighten, repeat the S.C.A.N. steps as often as needed.

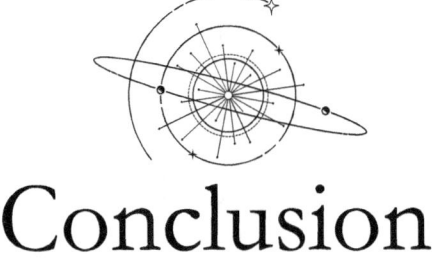

Conclusion

Embracing the natural cycles of life allows us to align with the rhythm of the Cosmos. For those living in the Southern and Northern Hemispheres, the changing seasons serve as powerful tools for manifestation. Our journeys follow similar patterns as nature goes through growth, transformation, and renewal phases. There is a time to plant seeds of intention, a time to take action, a time to harvest our efforts, and a time for rest and reflection. By honouring these cycles, we learn to trust in the divine timing of our manifestations and release the need for control.

I have created four dated workbooks to guide you through this process: Spring - Sow The Seeds Of Success, Summer - Cultivate Your Dreams, Autumn - Refine Your Vision, and Winter - Align Inner Transformation. Each workbook includes additional notes and a 13-week action plan, with some featuring weekly activities and others daily tasks. Each workbook also contains a ritual for each full moon, with the possibility of two full moons in a month (a Blue Moon). These workbooks invite you to trust the Cosmic rhythm and embrace the cyclical journey of becoming a new you.

As you stand on the threshold of this transformative journey, you are invited to surrender to the natural rhythm of the Cosmos. Trust that the growth, rest, and renewal cycles are designed to support your highest good just as the sun rises and sets. Embrace the cyclical journey of life, understanding that every season, phase, and moment has its purpose. The Cosmos always conspires in your favour, guiding you through the ebbs and flows of manifestation and growth. By leaning into this rhythm, you align yourself with divine timing, allowing your life to unfold in perfect harmony.

Remember, each season is a chapter in your story, a step toward self-discovery and fulfilment. Trust the journey, for it is uniquely yours, woven by the hands of the Cosmos itself.

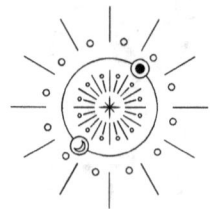

"Cosmic Flow invites you to dance with the rhythm of life"

Teanna

Reference Guides

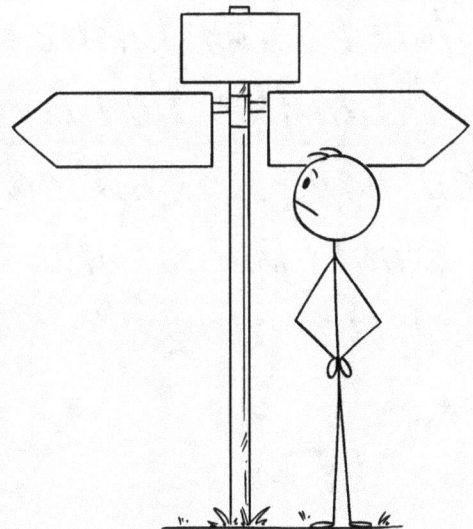

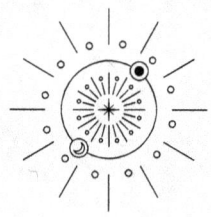

"A resolution is hoping for a better future. Manifestation is knowing it is already yours and acting accordingly"

Teanna ♡

New Year Resolutions Vs Manifestation

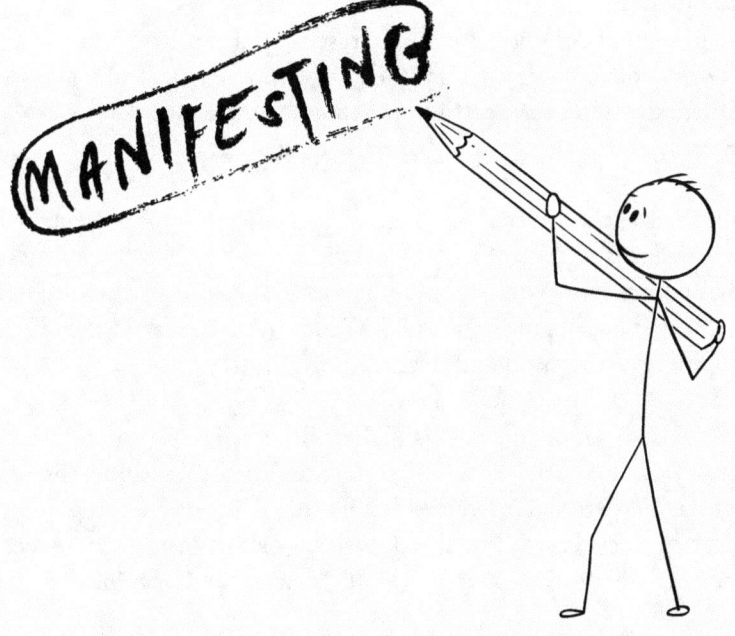

One key thing Cosmic energy can help with is manifesting abundance in all areas of life. But first, let me clarify the difference between resolutions (especially at New Year's and manifesting), as there is a big difference in the approach, mindset, and execution.

Resolutions are typically goal-oriented commitments that involve discipline, planning, and active effort. They are often framed as firm decisions to achieve a specific outcome, such as committing to the gym three times a week or saving a certain amount of money within a year. They are often framed as self-improvement or fixing something. Thus, resolutions rely heavily on willpower, structure, and external actions to create change, often requiring consistency and determination to achieve the desired results. These are often set in January when the Cosmic Energy is low. This double whammy of low Cosmic Energy and the need for willpower can lead to high failure rates, leading to feelings of disappointment and self-criticism, negatively impacting mental well-being.

 The Science

Research suggests that setting New Year's resolutions can have adverse effects on mental health, depending on how they are approached. While goal-setting can benefit motivation and self-improvement, unrealistic or overly rigid resolutions can lead to stress, anxiety, and decreased self-esteem.

A study published in the Journal of Clinical Psychology found that while about 40% of Americans set New Year's resolutions, only 8 - 20% successfully maintain them long-term. People who perceive their resolutions as 'unmet expectations' experience a drop in self-efficacy (the belief in the ability to succeed), leading to frustration and decreased motivation.

Additionally, "false hope syndrome" is higher. Researchers from the University of Toronto coined this term to describe the tendency to set unrealistic goals based on social or external pressures rather than intrinsic motivation. This often results in a cycle of initial enthusiasm, short-term adherence, and eventual failure, which can lead to guilt, shame, and diminished mental resilience.

However, people who frame their resolutions as 'intentions' focusing on progress rather than perfection tend to experience higher motivation, lower stress, and a greater sense of accomplishment. This is where manifestation comes in. It is more natural and based on aligning thoughts, emotions, actions and energy with a desired outcome. It focuses on visualisation, belief, aligned actions and attracting what you want by shifting your mindset and trusting the process.

From a psychological standpoint, manifestation encourages a mindset shift that reduces stress and enhances mental resilience. Studies on positive psychology and cognitive-behavioural therapy (CBT) suggest that focusing on gratitude, visualisation, and self-compassion increases neural pathways associated with emotional regulation and goal achievement, leading to lower anxiety and greater overall life satisfaction.

Additionally, research on circadian rhythms and seasonal cycles indicates that aligning actions with natural energy flows can enhance mental clarity, emotional stability, and long-term habit formation.

Therefore, practising manifestation in harmony with the natural flow of energy - particularly starting in March - aligns with biological, psychological, and environmental factors that support mental well-being.

While both approaches can be effective, manifestation tends to feel more fluid, natural, and in tune with the Cosmic energy flow.

The 'Cosmic Flow Method' is a balanced approach involving setting intentions through manifestation while taking practical steps to bring them to life.

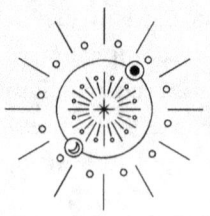

*"Everything is energy.
Match the frequency
of the reality you want,
and you cannot help
but get that reality."*

Attributed to Albert Einstein (though debated)*

Setting Intentions
REFERENCE GUIDE

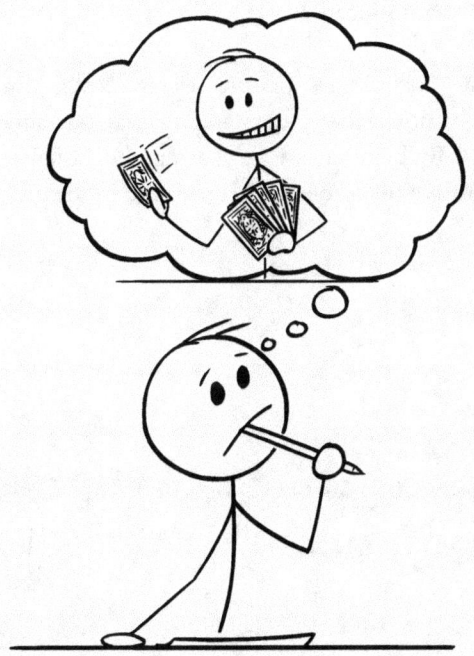

Negative intentions fall under the universal law of Karma. In simple terms, Karma is the universal law of cause and effect. It suggests that every action-good or bad- has consequences that will eventually return to the person who performed the action.

Karma works on a simple principle: Positive actions bring positive results, while negative actions bring negative results. If you do good deeds, show kindness, and act with good intentions, you will likely experience positive outcomes, such as happiness, success, or good fortune. Conversely, harmful actions, negative thoughts, or hurtful behaviours can lead to suffering, obstacles, or difficulties in the future.

There is often confusion about Karma. It is not about punishment or reward. Instead, a natural law of balance, much like gravity, helps maintain harmony in the Cosmos. Also, Karma is not instant. According to certain beliefs, manifesting can take time, sometimes even in future lives.

The idea of Karma encourages people to live ethically, responsibly, and compassionately. It promotes the understanding that our actions shape our lives and impact our world. By being aware of Karma, individuals can make conscious choices that create positive outcomes and contribute to the greater good.

So keep your intentions positive!

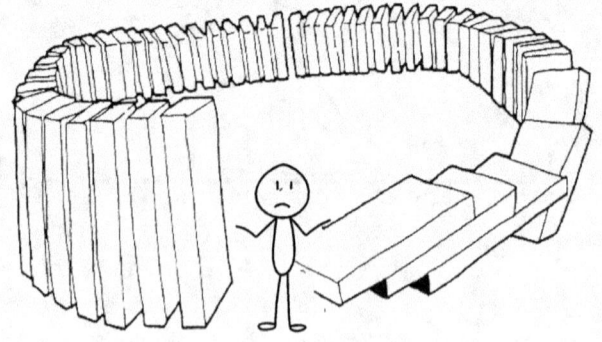

Negative intention examples are:

Control Over Others
Trying to manifest influence over some of your decisions, emotions, or actions go against free will and often lead to toxic relationships.

Material Greed Without Purpose
Manifesting excessive wealth or luxury only for selfish gain without gratitude or a desire to share abundance can lead to emptiness.

Jealousy and Comparison
Wishing for success to surpass or outshine others rather than for personal fulfilment brings insecurity and dissatisfaction.

Revenge and Harm
Manifesting negative outcomes for someone who wronged you creates a cycle of negativity and often rebounds in unexpected ways.

Fame and Recognition for Ego
Seeking attention and validation from others purely to feed an ego rather than for meaningful contribution, which can lead to shallow success.

Desperation and Neediness
Manifesting out of a place of lack or desperation (e.g., "I need this or I will be miserable") reinforces scarcity and fear.

Instant Gratification
Wanting immediate results without patience, hard work, or responsibility can lead to unsustainable or fleeting success.

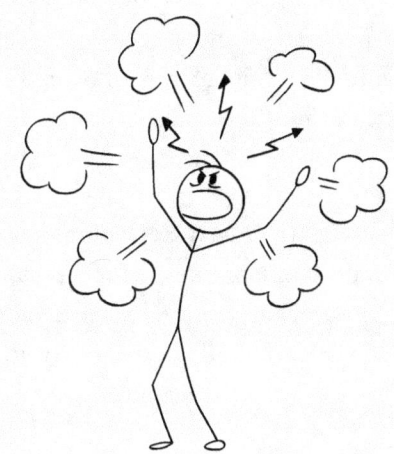

Seeking Validation
Manifesting success, beauty, or wealth solely to gain approval from others keeps you trapped in external validation rather than internal fulfilment.

Power and Domination
Wishing to be "better than" or to dominate others through status, influence, or control creates toxic dynamics and attracts conflict.

Dishonest Gain
Hoping for success, wealth, or opportunities through deception, manipulation, or unethical means often leads to long-term consequences.

Avoiding Accountability
Manifesting an escape from problems instead of personal growth and resolution can create a cycle of running from responsibilities.

Wishing for Others to Fail
Hoping competitors, ex-partners, or others struggle to make yourself look better breeds negativity and bad karma.

Superficial Beauty or Attraction
Wanting to manifest physical appearance changes purely for vanity or attention, without self-love, can lead to body image struggles.

Addiction to External Rewards
Manifesting money, fame, or status without emotional or spiritual fulfilment often results in emptiness despite material success.

Lust - Based Relationships
Wanting someone solely for their looks or physical attraction rather than a deep connection leads to shallow or toxic relationships.

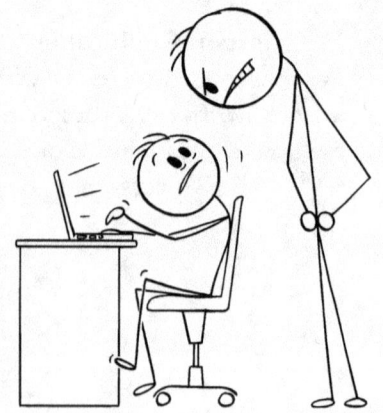

Positive intention examples are:

Personal Growth and Self - Love
Manifesting confidence, self - worth, and emotional resilience helps create a fulfilling life from within.

Abundance and Prosperity for All
Wishing for financial success while also desiring to uplift others ensures that wealth is shared and used for good.

Healing and Positivity
Manifesting good health, peace, and happiness for yourself and others foster a positive environment and attract uplifting energy.

Gratitude and Contentment
Manifesting appreciation for what you already have helps attract even more abundance and joy.

Confidence and Self - Worth
Affirming your own value and believing in yourself opens doors to opportunities and fulfilling experiences.

Forgiveness and Letting Go
Manifesting emotional freedom from past hurts allows you to move forward with peace and positivity.

Supportive and Loving Community
Attracting meaningful friendships and relationships that uplift and inspire you to create a fulfilling life.

Aligned Opportunities
Manifesting career, creative, or life opportunities that match your purpose and skills lead to greater satisfaction.

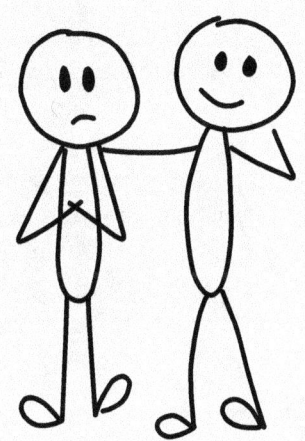

Joy and Playfulness
Calling in more fun, laughter, and lightheartedness helps create
a balanced and fulfilling life.

Generosity and Giving Back
Manifesting the ability to help others
whether through time, resources, or kindness - creates deeper fulfilment.

Healing from the Past
Releasing old wounds and manifesting emotional or physical
healing allows for a fresh start.

Strength and Resilience
Cultivating the ability to handle challenges with grace and perseverance
ensures long - term success.

Alignment with Your Higher Self
Manifesting clarity and guidance from your inner wisdom leads to
greater purpose and fulfilment.

Creativity and Inspiration
Attracting new ideas, artistic flow, and innovative thinking helps
with personal and professional growth.

Peaceful and Restful Sleep
Manifesting deep, restorative sleep improves overall well-being and energy.

Synchronicity and Divine Timing
Trusting that things will unfold at the right time reduces anxiety
and increases faith in the journey.

Strong Boundaries and Self - Respect
Calling in the confidence to say no to what does not serve you
and yes to what uplifts you.

Badly Written and Better Version of Intentions for Career and Success

Badly Written: I want a better job.
Better Version: I am attracting a fulfilling career that aligns with my passions, provides financial abundance, and allows me to grow professionally and personally.

Badly Written: I just want to be successful.
Better Version: I am creating success on my own terms, embracing opportunities, and consistently taking inspired action toward my goals.

Badly Written: I need more money.
Better Version: I am attracting wealth and financial abundance through my skills, talents, and the valuable contributions I make in my career.

Badly Written: I want a promotion.
Better Version: I am confidently stepping into leadership roles, demonstrating my value, and attracting well-deserved career advancements.

Badly Written: I do not want to struggle in my job anymore.
Better Version: I am thriving in a career that energizes me, challenges me to grow, and brings me joy and fulfillment every day.

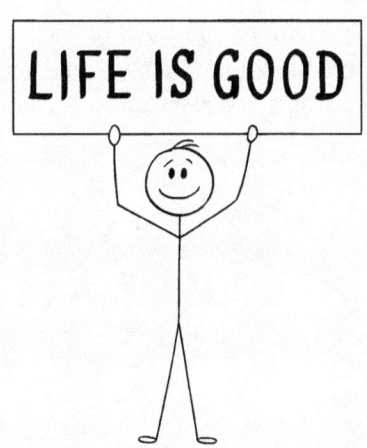

Badly Written and Better Version of Intentions for Love and Relationships

Badly Written: I want to find love.
Better Version: I am in a loving, healthy, and supportive relationship with a partner who values and respects me.

Badly Written: I do not want to be lonely anymore.
Better Version: I am surrounded by love and meaningful connections, attracting relationships that bring joy, support, and deep fulfillment into my life.

Badly Written: I hope someone loves me one day.
Better Version: I am worthy of love, and I attract a partner who cherishes, respects, and loves me unconditionally.

Badly Written: I just want my relationship to be better.
Better Version: My relationship is growing stronger every day as my partner and I communicate openly, love deeply, and support each other unconditionally.

Badly Written: I am tired of bad relationships.
Better Version: I attract and nurture healthy, loving, and harmonious relationships that align with my highest self and bring me happiness.

Badly Written and Better Version of Intentions for Money and Abundance

Badly Written: I want more money.
Better Version: I am financially abundant, and money flows to me effortlessly through multiple sources as I embrace opportunities for prosperity.

Badly Written: I need to stop struggling with money.
Better Version: I am financially secure, and abundance flows to me easily as I make wise financial decisions and attract prosperity.

Badly Written: I want to be rich.
Better Version: I am creating wealth through my talents, hard work, and smart investments, allowing me to live a life of freedom and abundance.

Badly Written: I just need a better job that pays more.
Better Version: I attract career opportunities that align with my skills and passions, providing financial abundance and professional growth.

Badly Written: I am tired of living paycheck to paycheck
Better Version: I am open to new income streams and financial growth, and I effortlessly attract wealth and opportunities that support my abundant lifestyle.

Badly Written and Better Version of Intentions for Health and Well-Being

Badly Written: I want to be healthier.
Better Version: I am vibrant, strong, and full of energy, nourishing my body with healthy choices and balanced habits every day.

Badly Written: I need to lose weight.
Better Version: I honor my body by nourishing it with healthy foods, staying active, and embracing a balanced lifestyle that supports my well-being.

Badly Written: I do not want to feel tired all the time.
Better Version: My body is full of energy, and I wake up each day feeling refreshed, revitalised, and ready to thrive.

Badly Written: I just want to stop getting sick.
Better Version: My body is strong, resilient, and in perfect harmony, naturally healing and protecting itself with ease.

Badly Written: I wish I had more motivation to be healthy.
Better Version: I am committed to my health and well-being, making choices that strengthen my body, uplift my mind, and energize my spirit every day.

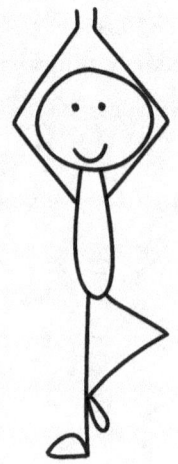

Learning Style Self-Check Quiz

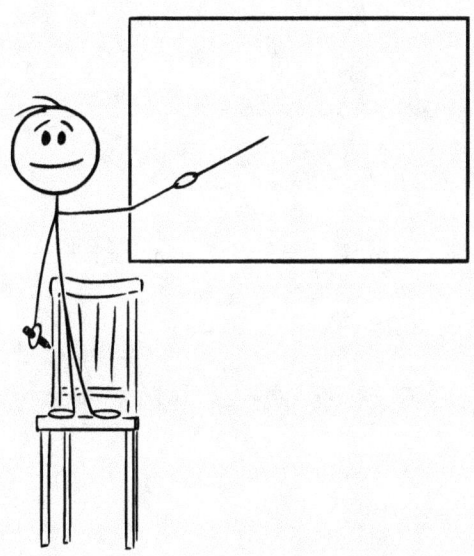

Just answer each question and keep track of how many times you choose A, B, C, or D. Your dominant learning style will be revealed at the end!

1. When trying to remember something, you usually...
A) Picture it in your mind
B) Say it out loud or repeat it in your head
C) Write it down or read over your notes
D) Try to act it out or physically do something with it

2. In a class or seminar, you prefer...
A) Diagrams, charts, or slides
B) Lectures, discussions, and podcasts
C) Reading handouts or written guides
D) Hands-on activities or group projects

3. When learning a new skill, what helps most?
A) Watching a video or looking at pictures
B) Hearing someone explain it step-by-step
C) Reading instructions or writing notes
D) Trying it yourself and learning by doing

4. Which of these tools excites you most for manifesting?
A) Vision boards and Pinterest mood boards
B) Guided meditations, affirmations, or music
C) Journalling, scripting, or making a plan
D) Dancing, moving, or physically stepping into your "future self"

5. How do you best express how you feel?
A) Drawing, doodling, or using visuals
B) Talking it out or using voice notes
C) Writing in a journal or texting someone
D) Through body language, gestures, or movement

Results: Tally your answers!

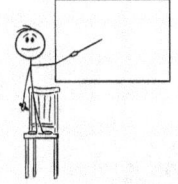

Mostly A = Visual Learner
You learn best by seeing - use visualisation, images, vision boards, and colours to evoke emotion and manifest powerfully.

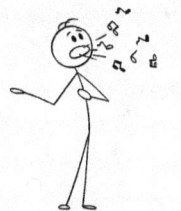

Mostly B = Auditory Learner
you are tuned in to sound - try spoken affirmations, voice notes, meditations, and music to align emotionally.

Mostly C = Reading/Writing Learner
Words are your strength - scripting, journalling, and reading meaningful content will help you manifest with clarity and emotion.

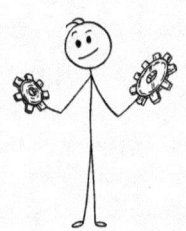

Mostly D = Kinaesthetic Learner
You thrive through doing - use movement, embodiment, rituals, and hands-on techniques to connect emotionally to your vision.

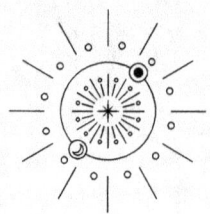

"In stillness, we become one with the cosmos - a quiet pulse in the heart of the universe."

Teanna

Meditation and Chakras
REFERENCE GUIDE

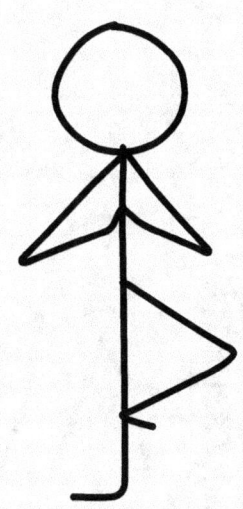

Chakras

These are your energy centres, which extend beyond your physical presence. They are seen as non-physical, spinning wheels of energy within your subtle body and are often artistically represented as lotus flowers.

Seven main energy centres (Chakras) are observed in many Eastern spiritual and healing practices, including Hinduism, Buddhism, and Yoga. The concept of chakras has also influenced Western practices such as psychology and complementary medicine through Reiki and Meditation.

There are various ways to work with your energy and chakras, from using crystals for balance to Reiki and Ayurvedic practices. But in all cases, we control these energy points via our thoughts, actions, and experiences in life. It easily flows when this energy is linked to the Cosmic energy cycles.

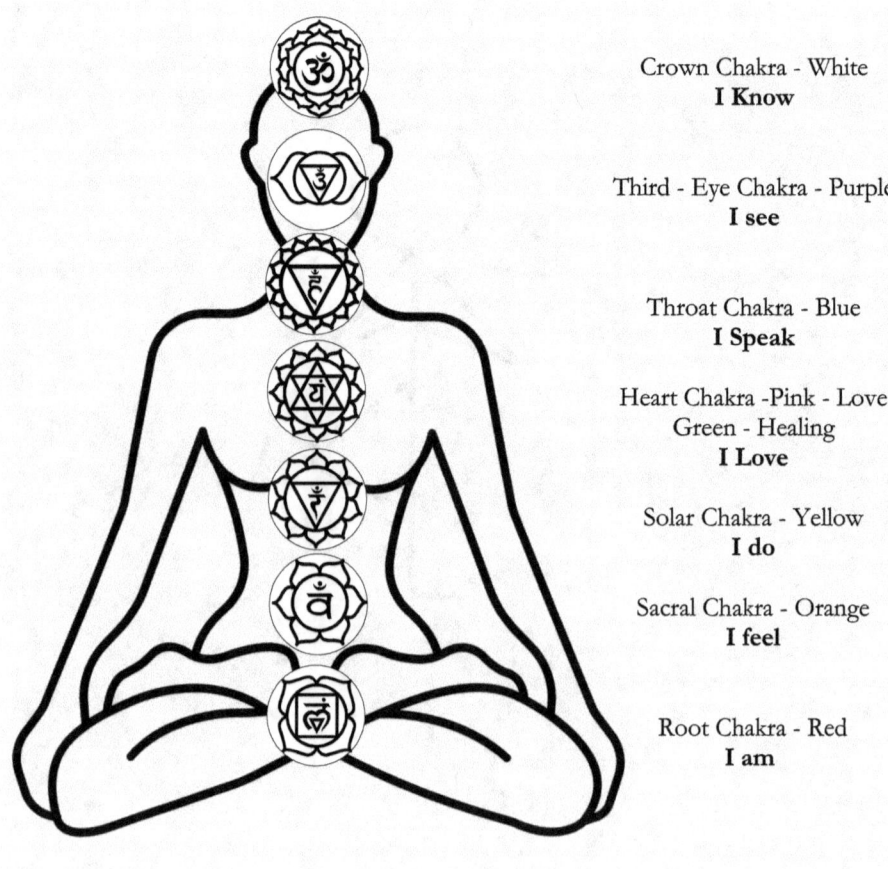

Crown Chakra - White
I Know

Third - Eye Chakra - Purple
I see

Throat Chakra - Blue
I Speak

Heart Chakra -Pink - Love
Green - Healing
I Love

Solar Chakra - Yellow
I do

Sacral Chakra - Orange
I feel

Root Chakra - Red
I am

The chakras represent various aspects of our being, each associated with different emotions, elements, and functions. Starting from the top, the " crown' chakra is linked to divine wisdom, imagination, and spirituality - following, the 'third eye' chakra centres on intuition, insight, and dreams. The ' throat' chakra emphasises expression, truth, leadership, and fluid communication.

The heart chakra embodies compassion, love, and connection to oneself and others. The solar plexus chakra, often called the power chakra, deals with personal power, self-confidence, and a sense of control. The sacral chakra focuses on emotions, creativity, and body confidence. Finally, the root chakra is connected to security, survival instincts, and foundational beliefs around money.

Focusing on a particular chakra during meditation can help deepen your meditative experience, fostering a sense of balance and well-being.

The Science
The human body generates measurable energy in the form of electromagnetic fields. For example, the electrical activity of the heart (measured by an electrocardiogram, or ECG) and the brain (measured by an electroencephalogram, or EEG) are well - documented phenomena in modern medicine. These fields arise from the bioelectrical signals that our organs and cells produce.

However, when it comes to the idea of a subtle energy field or aura, modern science lacks the tools to measure this subtle energy. Therefore, the scientific evidence is much less clear. In contrast, some alternative techniques, such as Kirlian photography, claim to capture these energy fields, such methods have not been widely accepted or validated by the mainstream scientific community. Thus, while measurable electromagnetic energy exists around the body, the broader claims about subtle energies that extend beyond these known physical phenomena remain unproven by current scientific standards. But this does not mean they are not there, and as you can connect further to energy, you will start to feel it.

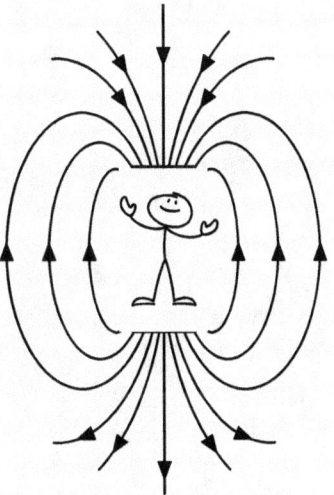

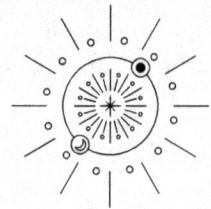

"Sound is the bridge between the seen and unseen -it carries intention, shifts energy, and speaks the language of the soul."

Unknown

Sound Frequencies
REFERENCE GUIDE

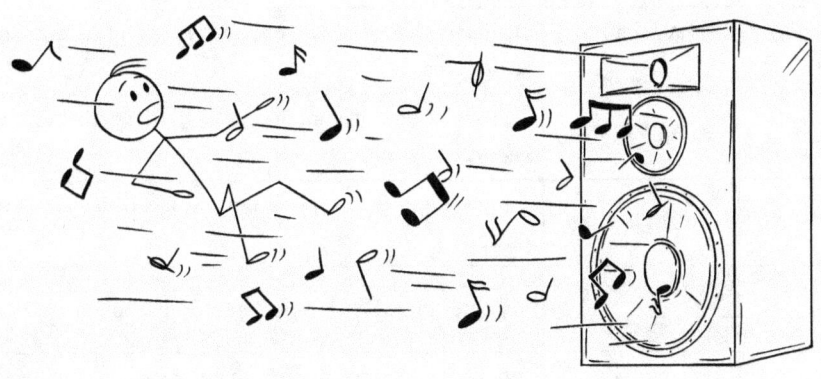

Frequency (Hz)	Name	Purpose in Manifestation
111	Holy Frequency	Induces deep meditation, promotes clarity, and aligns with higher self.
144	Ascension Frequency	Enhances spiritual awakening, activates higher consciousness, and connects with divine wisdom.
174	Healing Frequency	Reduces pain, relieves stress, and promotes healing.
222	Balance Frequency	Enhances equilibrium, stability, and manifestation of desires.
285	Regeneration Frequency	Helps with tissue healing, cellular regeneration, and emotional balance.
333	Ascended Masters Frequency	Connects with divine guidance and amplifies spiritual growth.
396	Liberation Frequency	Releases fear, guilt, and subconscious blockages.
417	Transformation Frequency	Facilitates change, removes negative energy, and clears past trauma.
432	Natural Frequency	Aligns with nature, enhances relaxation, and brings emotional harmony.
440	Standard Tuning	Common in modern music but can feel disharmonious to some.
528	Love Frequency	Promotes love, DNA repair, and transformation.
639	Connection Frequency	Enhances relationships, communication, and connection with others.
741	Detox Frequency	Cleanses the mind, body, and spirit; removes toxins and negativity.
852	Awakening Frequency	Expands consciousness, enhances intuition, and deepens spiritual awareness.
963	Divine Frequency	Connects to higher consciousness, enlightenment, and the Cosmos.

Frequency (Hz)	Name	Purpose in Manifestation
999	Completion Frequency	Signifies the end of a cycle, new beginnings, and spiritual enlightenment.
444	Angelic Frequency	Aligns with angelic energies, enhances protection, and supports healing.
555	Change Frequency	Encourages transformation, new beginnings, and breaking old patterns.
666	Harmonisation Frequency	Balances mind, body, and spirit (despite negative associations).
777	Luck Frequency	Attracts divine guidance, luck, and spiritual awakening.
888	Abundance Frequency	Manifests financial prosperity, success, and infinite energy.

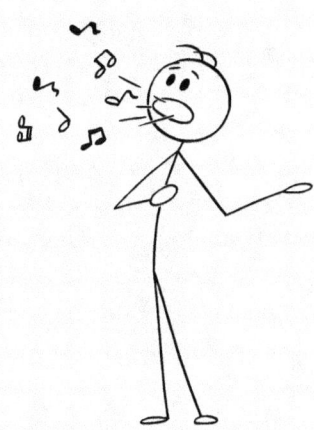

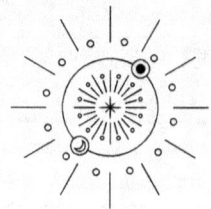

"Numbers are the language of the cosmos - each one carries a frequency, a vibration, a key to unlock hidden energy within and around us."

Unknown

Frequency of Numbers
REFERENCE GUIDE

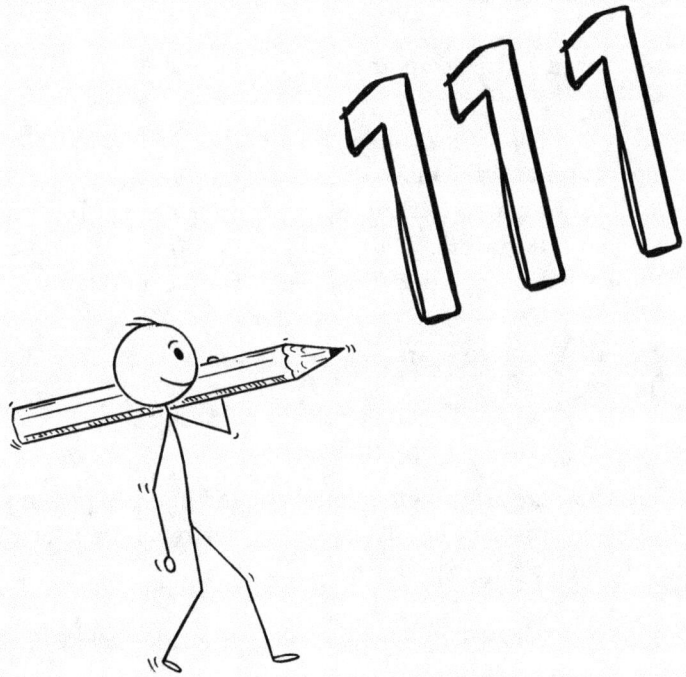

Numerology

Numerology suggests that numbers have powerful vibrational energy that can influence our lives. Each number holds a unique meaning and can help us better understand our personalities, challenges, and strengths. Whether through core numbers, master numbers, or angel numbers, numerology offers guidance for personal growth and self-discovery.

Many people notice repeated numbers when synchronicities are about to happen, and each has a message to convey.

Core Numbers (0-9) and Their Meanings
These single-digit numbers form the foundation of numerology. Every other number can be reduced to one of these by adding its digits together.

Number 1 - Leadership and New Beginnings
The number 1 represents independence, ambition, and originality. It symbolises a pioneering spirit, innovation, and self-confidence. People associated with this number are often strong leaders and risk-takers.

For example, those with a Life Path Number 1 are natural leaders who enjoy taking initiative.

Number 2 - Cooperation and Balance
The number 2 symbolises harmony, relationships, and diplomacy. It represents sensitivity, patience, and teamwork. This number is often associated with peacemakers and those who value partnership and emotional connections.

People with a Life Path Number 2 are usually kind, empathetic, and great at working with others.

Number 3 - Creativity and Expression
The number 3 is linked to creativity, communication, and joy. It represents self-expression, optimism, and artistic ability. Those with this number often have a gift for words, whether through writing, speaking, or the arts.

A person with a Life Path Number 3 is typically social, charismatic, and full of creative energy.

Number 4 - Stability and Hard Work

The number 4 represents discipline, structure, and practicality. It is the number of builders, planners, and hardworking individuals who focus on creating solid foundations. People with this number are reliable and prefer order and security.

For instance, those with a Life Path Number 4 are often determined, logical, and persistent in their goals.

Number 5 - Freedom and Change

The number 5 symbolises adventure, curiosity, and adaptability. It represents people who crave freedom, excitement, and variety in life. Those influenced by this number are often travellers, risk-takers, and highly adaptable to new situations.

A person with a Life Path Number 5 thrives on change and dislikes routines.

Number 6 - Love and Responsibility

The number 6 is associated with family, compassion, and nurturing. It represents care giving, responsibility, and unconditional love. People influenced by this number often feel a strong need to protect and support others.

For example, a person with a Life Path Number 6 is naturally caring and tends to prioritise relationships and family life.

Number 7 - Spirituality and Intuition

The number 7 symbolises wisdom, introspection, and spiritual awareness. It is the number of deep thinkers, philosophers, and seekers of truth. People associated with this number often have strong intuition and a desire to explore life's mysteries.

Those with a Life Path Number 7 are usually analytical, reflective, and drawn to spiritual or intellectual pursuits.

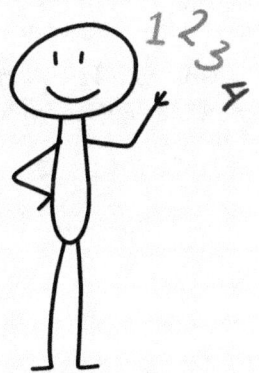

Number 8 - Power and Success

The number 8 represents authority, financial success, and material achievement. It is the number of business-minded, ambitious, and disciplined individuals who strive for prosperity and influence.

For example, a person with a Life Path Number 8 is often focused on career growth, financial success, and leadership roles.

Number 9 - Humanitarianism and Wisdom
The number 9 symbolises compassion, wisdom, and humanitarian efforts. It represents people who are generous, selfless, and driven by a desire to help others.

A person with a Life Path Number 9 often feels a strong sense of purpose and seeks to make a positive impact on the world.

Number 0 - Infinite Potential
The number 0 represents infinity, wholeness, and spiritual potential. It amplifies the energy of any number it appears with and symbolises the connection between the material and spiritual worlds.

Master Numbers (11, 22, 33)
In numerology, some numbers are considered Master Numbers because they hold a higher spiritual significance and greater potential.

Number 11 - Intuition and Enlightenment
11 is a powerful number associated with spiritual insight, intuition, and enlightenment. It represents people who are highly sensitive, visionary, and deeply connected to their inner wisdom.

Those with a Life Path Number 11 often experience heightened intuition and a strong desire to inspire and uplift others.

Number 22 - The Master Builder
The number 22, known as the Master Builder, symbolises great potential, success, and practicality. It represents people who can turn dreams into reality through discipline and effort.

A person with Life Path Number 22 has the ability to create lasting legacies and significantly influence the world.

Number 33 - The Master Teacher

The number 33 is considered the Master Teacher and represents unconditional love, wisdom, and spiritual guidance. It symbolises healing, nurturing, and a deep desire to help others.

Those with a Life Path Number 33 often serve as mentors, healers, or guides who bring light and wisdom to the world.

How to Calculate Your Life Path Number

Your Life Path Number is the most important number in numerology. It reveals your personality, strengths, challenges, and life purpose. To calculate your Life

Path Number, follow these steps:

Step 1: Write down your full birth date

For example, if you were born on March 29, 1995 (03/29/1995)

Step 2: Add all the digits together

$0 + 3 + 2 + 9 + 1 + 9 + 9 + 5 = 38$

Step 3: Reduce to a single digit

$3 + 8 = 11$

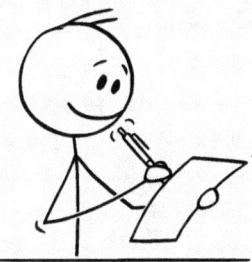

Since 11 is a Master Number, we do not reduce it further. If the final number is 11, 22, or 33, it remains a Master Number.

If the sum is not a Master Number, continue reducing until you reach a single digit.

Angel Numbers and Their Meanings

Angel numbers are repeated number sequences that carry divine messages.

111 - New Beginnings and Manifestation
Seeing 111 is a sign that your thoughts are manifesting quickly. It encourages you to stay focused on positive intentions.

222 - Balance and Harmony
The number 222 reminds us to stay patient and trust that everything aligns. It symbolises harmony in relationships and life.

333 - Creativity and Divine Support
Seeing 333 means that the Cosmos are guiding your creativity. It is a sign of encouragement from spiritual forces.

444 - Protection and Stability
The number 444 signifies that your angels or guides are protecting you. It symbolises strength, security, and support.

555 - Change and Transformation
Seeing 555 means that a significant change is coming.

It is a sign to embrace new opportunities and trust the process.

666 - Self-Reflection and Balance
Despite its negative reputation, 666 symbolises the need to refocus on spiritual and emotional balance rather than material worries.

Shadow Work

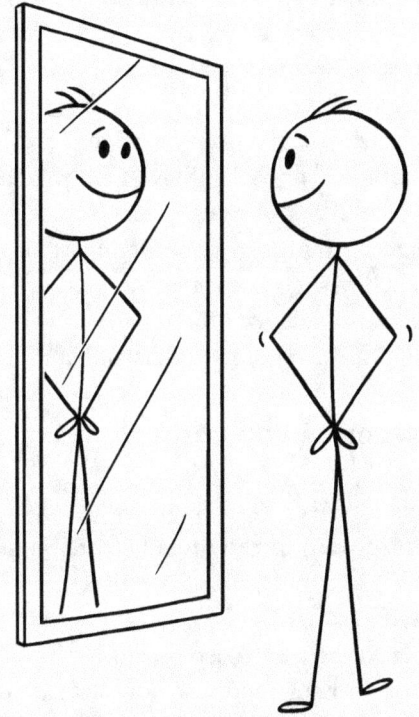

Shadow work is the process of exploring the unconscious parts of yourself - traits, emotions, and desires you may have rejected or hidden. It involves acknowledging and accepting these "shadow" aspects instead of ignoring or suppressing them. By doing shadow work, you can heal emotional wounds, break negative patterns, and grow into a more whole, authentic version of yourself.

Doing shadow work is a personal and introspective process. I cover this in the winter workbook, but here are a few ways to start:

1. Self-reflection – Notice strong emotional reactions, triggers, or judgments you have toward others. These can be clues to your shadow.
2. Journaling – Write honestly about your fears, insecurities, regrets, and thoughts you usually hide. Let it all out without judgment.
3. Inner child work – Revisit your past and connect with your version of feeling rejected, shamed, or silenced.
4. Meditation – Quiet your mind and observe what surfaces – thoughts or feelings you usually suppress.
5. Shadow prompts – Ask yourself deep questions like, "What parts of myself do I try to hide from others?" or "When have I felt jealous, ashamed, or resentful, and why?"
6. Therapy or guidance – Working with a therapist or coach who understands shadow work can help you go deeper safely.
7. Compassion: Accept and integrate these parts of yourself without shame. The goal is not to get rid of them but to understand and make peace with them.

Shadow work exercises you can try on your own

Shadow Work Exercise: "Meet Your Shadow"
Goal: To explore a part of yourself you often hide, reject, or feel ashamed of.

Step 1: Ground Yourself
- Sit somewhere quiet. Take a few deep breaths.
- Close your eyes for a minute and just notice what you are feeling physically and emotionally.

Step 2: Identify a Trigger
- Consider a recent situation where you felt a strong emotional reaction (anger, jealousy, shame, etc.).
- Ask yourself:
- "What specifically bothered me about that moment or person?"

Step 3: Dig Deeper
- Now, write answers to these prompts in your journal:
  - What did I feel in that moment?
  - What did that situation say about me, deep down? (Example: "It made me feel like I am not good enough.")
  - Is there a part of me I try to hide from others? What is it?
  - Where did I learn that this part of me was unacceptable? Childhood? School? Society?
  - What would it feel like to accept this part of me, even just a little?

Step 4: Talk to the Shadow
- Imagine this rejected part of you as a younger version of yourself.
- Write a short letter to it. Say something like:
- "I see you. I understand why you feel this way. You were trying to protect me. You are allowed to be here."

Step 5: Breathe and Reflect
- Retake a few breaths and thank yourself for doing this work.
- Notice how you feel now - lighter, resistant, emotional - it is all okay.
- You can repeat this exercise regularly, each time with a new trigger or emotion.

2. The Mirror Exercise
- Look into a mirror for 2–5 minutes. Maintain soft eye contact.
- As you look at yourself, say things you usually avoid or hide. Example: "I see the part of me that's afraid of being unlovable." "I accept the part of me that wants to be in control."

Why it works: Facing your reflection directly activates deep emotions and brings your shadow forward for acknowledgement.

3. "The People You Judge" Journal Prompt
- Write down 3 people who trigger or annoy you.
- Then for each, write: "I dislike them because..." "This might reflect a part of me that..." Example:"I dislike how she always seeks attention." → "Maybe part of me is afraid to be seen, or envies that freedom."

4. Dialogue with Your Shadow
- Imagine a conversation between "You" and a shadow part. Example: If your shadow is "The Perfectionist," have a back-and-forth chat in your journal:
- You: Why are you always pushing me?
- Shadow: Because if I stop, you'll be judged or fail.
- End with: "What do you need from me?"

5. Art as Shadow Expression
Take some paper and just draw or paint how you feel - especially when you are in a triggered or raw state.
do not try to make it pretty or meaningful. Let your hand move intuitively.
Afterwards, reflect on what came out and what it might say about your hidden emotions.

6. Write Your "Dark Side" Bio
- Write a fictional, exaggerated version of yourself - all the parts you normally hide or deny.
- Let the voice be raw, sarcastic, proud, honest. Example: "I crave validation. I manipulate to feel secure. I judge because I am scared of being judged."
- Then reflect: Which parts of this are true? Which parts need compassion?

7. "I Am Both" Statements
- Write statements that integrate both your light and shadow.
- Examples:
    - "I am both kind and selfish."
    - "I am both confident and insecure."
    - "I am both loving and angry."
    - This helps reduce the shame around being complex and human.

Dream Work

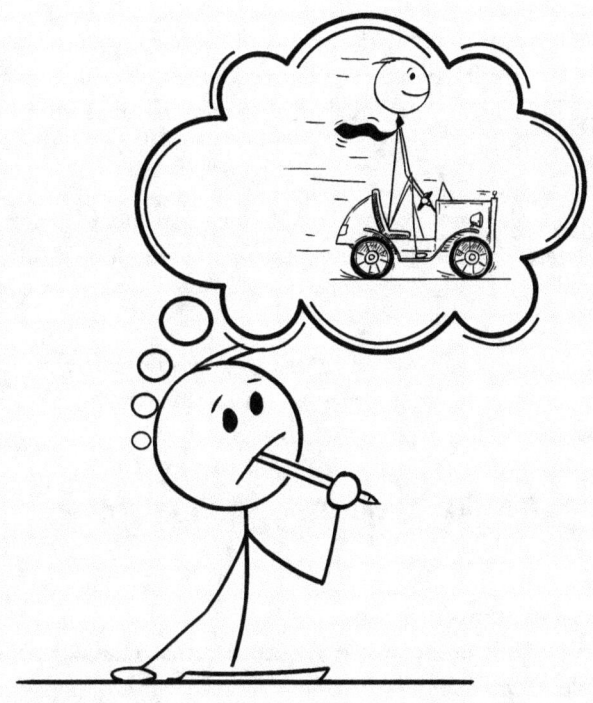

"Dreamwork" refers to the process of exploring, analysing, and interpreting dreams to gain insight into the subconscious mind. It is often used in therapy, spirituality, and personal development.

Dreamwork is vital in psychology and therapy, especially in Freudian and Jungian traditions. Sigmund Freud believed dreams express repressed desires, and his dream work method involved uncovering hidden meanings through symbols. Carl Jung, on the other hand, saw dreams as reflections of the unconscious that could guide personal growth. His approach focused on identifying archetypes, symbols, and recurring patterns.

In spiritual or shamanic practices, dreams are often viewed as messages from spirit guides, ancestors, or the higher self. Dreamwork in this context might include dream journaling, lucid dreaming, or rituals meant to receive guidance.

In personal development, dream work is used to understand emotions, solve problems, or inspire creativity. This often involves keeping a dream journal or participating in group dream-sharing circles to explore themes and patterns in dreams.

Some people also use dream work to develop lucid dreaming skills, where they become aware that they are dreaming and intentionally interact with the dream world.

Here is a simple but powerful dream work and manifestation exercise that blends intention setting, dream journaling, and visualisation. You can do this at night before bed and in the morning when you wake up.

Manifesting Through Dream Work – Daily Exercise
Before Bed (10–15 minutes)

- Set an Intention (2–3 mins):
    - Sit quietly and take a few deep breaths. Think about one thing you would like to manifest
    - Say out loud or write: "Tonight, I invite my dreams to guide me toward [insert what you want to manifest]. I am open to signs, messages, and inspiration."

Visualisation (5 mins):
- Close your eyes and imagine your desired outcome as if it is already real. Picture it in vivid detail - what does it look, sound, and feel like? Let yourself feel the joy, peace, or excitement of it.

Dream Journal by Your Bed:
- Keep a notebook and pen beside your bed. The moment you wake up, be ready to jot down any dreams or images. Even a single word or feeling is worth capturing.

Morning (5–10 minutes)
Write Down Your Dreams:
- When you wake up before your logical brain kicks in, write down anything you remember from your dreams. Do not worry if it does not make sense. Symbols and fragments are still meaningful.

Reflect:
- Ask yourself: Did anything in the dream connect to my intention? What might this dream be trying to tell me? Write a few lines of reflection.

Affirmation for the Day:
- Create an affirmation based on your intention or dream. For example: "I am in alignment with new opportunities."
- Say it a few times as you start your day.

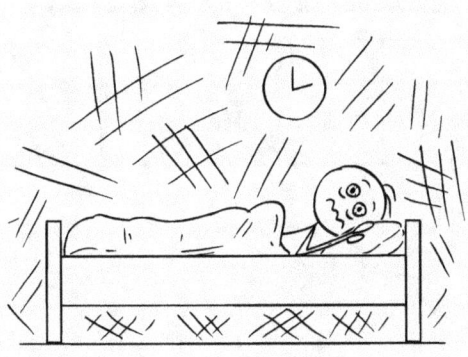

Pomodoro Technique

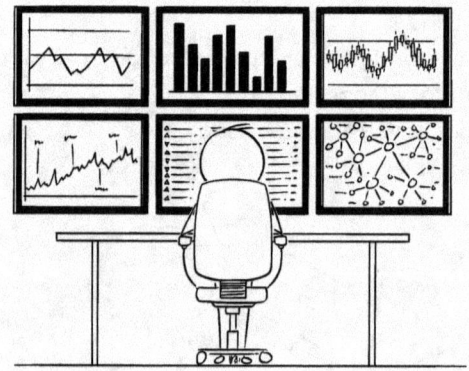

The Pomodoro Technique is a time management method developed by Francesco Cirillo in the late 1980s. It uses a timer to break work into intervals, typically:

25 minutes of focused work
5-minute break

After four "Pomodoro's," take a longer break (15–30 minutes)

The idea is that short bursts of focus help keep your mind fresh and productive while reducing burnout and procrastination.

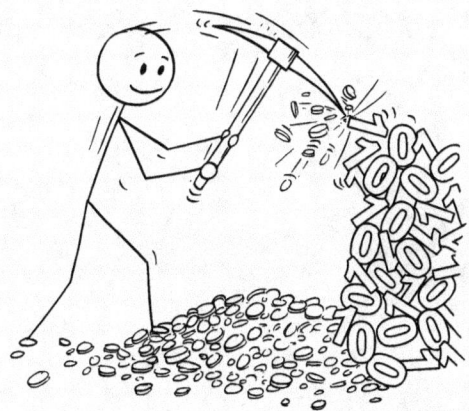

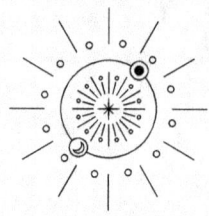

"Coaching is unlocking a person's potential to maximize their own performance. It is helping them to learn rather than teaching them."

Sir John Whitmore

Inner Critic Vs Inner Coach

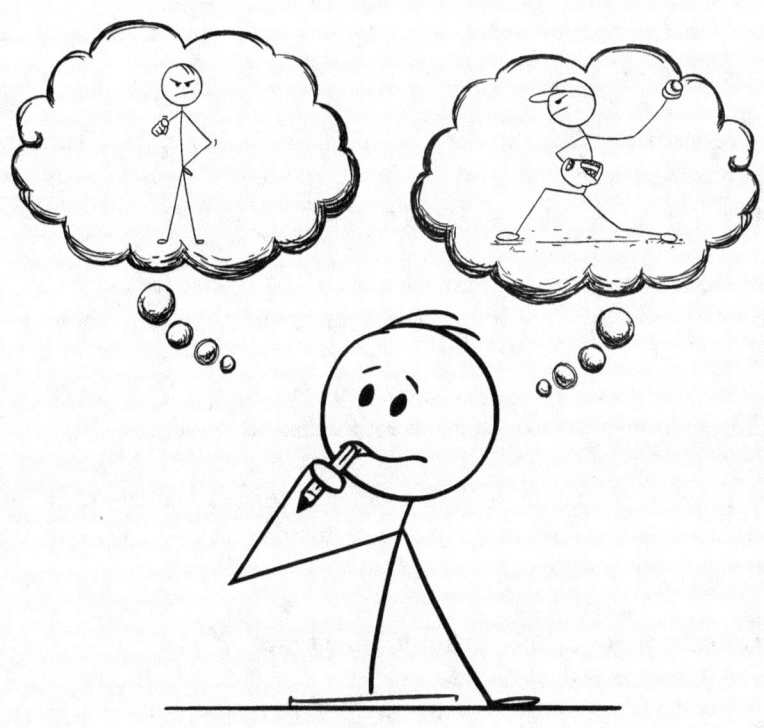

The inner critic and the inner coach are distinct voices in our inner dialogue. Understanding their differences can significantly impact how we relate to ourselves, especially regarding personal growth, creativity, and self-confidence.

The inner critic is that harsh, judgmental voice in your mind that often tells you you are not good enough, that you will fail, or that you should not even try. It might say, "You always mess things up," or "Who do you think you are to do this?" While it often stems from a protective place - trying to shield you from failure or rejection - it tends to hold you back and erode your confidence. This voice is usually shaped by past experiences, fears, or criticisms that you have internalised over time.

In contrast, the inner coach is supportive, compassionate, and realistic. It encourages you to keep going even when things are tough. It might say, "This is challenging, but you have faced hard things before," or "You made a mistake - let us learn from it and grow." The inner coach acknowledges obstacles but believes in your ability to overcome them. It speaks with kindness, wisdom, and resilience, helping you move forward rather than stay stuck.

The key difference between the two lies in their tone and impact. The inner critic focuses on flaws and fears, while the inner coach focuses on growth and possibility. One keeps you small, and the other helps you rise.

To shift from your inner critic to your inner coach, start by noticing when the critical voice appears. To create some distance, give it a name like "The Perfectionist" or "Doom Voice." Then ask yourself, "What would my inner coach say right now?" With practice, you can strengthen the coach's voice and turn your inner dialogue into a source of support rather than self-sabotage.

Here is a simple and effective Mini Journaling Practice to help shift from your inner critic to your inner coach. You can do this daily or whenever you catch yourself being self-critical.

Inner Critic to Inner Coach – Mini Journal Practice
1. What did my inner critic say today?
Write down the exact thought or phrase. Be honest. Example: "I'll never get this right. I am not good enough."

- How did it make me feel?

Notice and name the emotions that came up. Example: "I felt anxious, discouraged, and small."

- Where might this voice be coming from?

Reflect for a moment - does this voice remind you of a past experience or person? Example: "It sounds like the pressure I felt in school to be perfect."

- What would my inner coach say instead?

Re frame the thought with compassion, honesty, and encouragement. Example: "It is okay not to get it perfect the first time. I am learning, and that's what matters."

- What small step can I take today to move forward?

End with an action or mindset shift. Example: "I'll give it another try and focus on progress, not perfection."

You can keep this as a daily template in a notebook or notes app. Just 5 minutes a day can slowly retrain your inner voice to be your biggest ally.

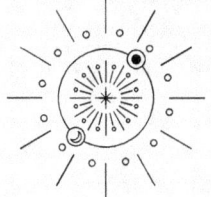

"The longest conversation you will ever have is the one you have with yourself. Make it kind. Make it true. Make it worth listening to."

Teanna

Not everyone has an inner voice

Do not worry if you cannot hear an inner dialogue; not everyone experiences an inner voice in the same way.

While many people have an internal monologue - a voice that narrates thoughts, makes decisions, or rehearses conversations - others think differently. Some process thoughts through images, abstract concepts, physical sensations, or emotions rather than verbal language. Research shows that inner experience is highly individual, and not everyone consistently hears a verbal internal monologue.

This variation can be influenced by factors like personality, neurodiversity (such as autism, ADHD, or aphantasia), and cultural background. For example, people with aphantasia may lack inner imagery and an internal voice, while others might have rich internal experiences filled with dialogue and visuals. Estimates suggest that around 25% to 30% of people regularly experience a constant inner monologue, while about 5% to 10% report having no inner monologue. The remaining 60% to 70% fall somewhere in between, experiencing an internal voice sometimes, often blended with other forms of thinking.

Regardless of how it shows up, there is no right or wrong way to think and process information through our own unique cognitive patterns. Therefore, we should use the appropriate tools to manifest and make changes.

How to Hack Your Brain
REFERENCE GUIDE

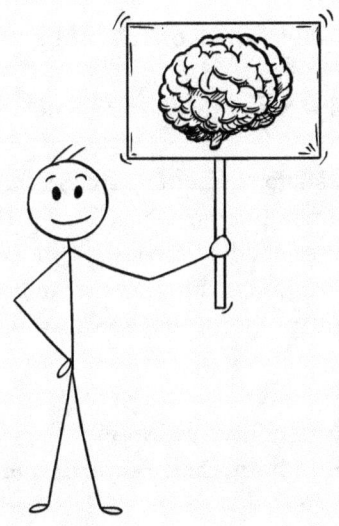

Create chemical reactions to come to
emotional balance quicker

The brain is a complex biochemical system that relies on various neurotransmitters, hormones, and other chemicals to regulate mood, cognition, memory, and bodily functions. "Hacking" your brain chemistry involves using natural, science-backed methods to optimise these neurotransmitters, hormones, and other brain chemicals for improved mood, focus, motivation, and overall well-being.

Neurotransmitters (Chemical Messengers)
These are chemicals that transmit signals between neurons. They play key roles in mood, behaviour, learning, and memory.
- Excitatory Neurotransmitters (Stimulating Brain Activity)
- Glutamate - The most abundant excitatory neurotransmitter, essential for learning, memory, and brain function.
- Dopamine - associated with pleasure, motivation, reward, and movement.
- Norepinephrine (Noradrenaline) - Enhances alertness, attention, and the body's stress response.
- Epinephrine (Adrenaline) - Involved in the "fight or flight" response, increasing heart rate and alertness.
- Acetylcholine (ACh) - Supports learning, memory, attention, and muscle activation.
- Inhibitory Neurotransmitters (Calming Brain Activity)
- GABA (Gamma-aminobutyric acid) - The primary inhibitory neurotransmitter that calms the nervous system and reduces anxiety.
- Serotonin - Regulates mood, sleep, appetite, and emotional stability.
- Glycine - Helps regulate motor and sensory functions, particularly in the spinal cord.

Neurohormones (Brain - Produced Hormones)
These chemicals function as hormones and neurotransmitters, influencing brain and body processes.
- Oxytocin - Known as the "love hormone," fosters bonding, trust, and social connections.
- Vasopressin - Regulates water balance and blood pressure and plays a role in bonding and memory.
- Cortisol - The stress hormone that prepares the body for challenges but can lead to anxiety if chronically high.
- Melatonin controls sleep and wake cycles and is influenced by light exposure.

- Endorphins - Natural painkillers that also promote pleasure and well-being.

Neuromodulators (Regulators of Neurotransmitter Activity)
- These chemicals fine-tune the effects of neurotransmitters over a broader area of the brain.

Endocannabinoids (Anandamide and 2 - AG) - Regulate mood, appetite, pain, and memory.
- Substance P - Involved in pain perception and inflammation.
- Neuropeptide Y (NPY) - Regulates stress, anxiety, and hunger.

Other Brain Chemicals
- Nitric Oxide (NO) - A gas that acts as a neurotransmitter, regulating blood flow and memory formation.
- Histamine - Plays a role in wakefulness, immune response, and appetite control.
- Lactic Acid - Produced during brain activity and helps with energy metabolism.

Hormones That Affect Brain Function
While produced outside the brain, these hormones influence brain activity:
- Testosterone and Estrogen - Affects mood, memory, and cognitive functions.
- Thyroid Hormones (T3 and T4) - Control metabolism and energy levels in the brain.
- Insulin - Regulates blood sugar and plays a role in brain function and neuroplasticity.
- Prolactin - Involved in reproductive behaviors, stress, and immune function.

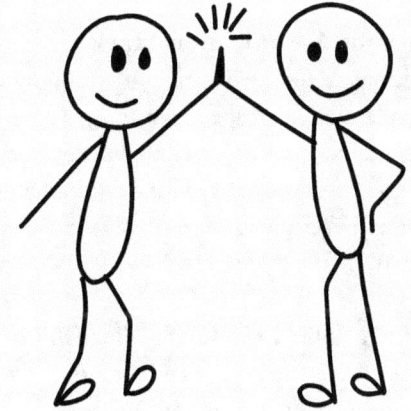

Dopamine

This is the brain's "reward" chemical for motivation, reward, pleasure, and focus. You can get a quick dopamine reset by engaging in physical triggers, such as a cold shower, which shocks your nervous system and boosts dopamine by up to 250%. Sunlight Exposure (vitamin D) also increases dopamine receptors naturally, and exercise, especially HIIT and weightlifting, but even 10 minutes of movement, i.e., jumping jacks, dancing, or walking, can give you a quick dopamine reset.

To get micro Dopamine hits, **Celebrate Small Wins, i.e.**, break big tasks into tiny steps and celebrate each one. The actual act of checking off a to-do list triggers dopamine, as does saying, "Good job, I did it!" after completing something, no matter how small.

Use the 'Temptation Bundling' Trick. This is where you pair a fun activity with a boring one. For example, listen to your favourite podcast while working out or watch a show while folding laundry, and your brain will start linking pleasure to the task!

Use the **Gamification Hack** - where you Make Things a Game by turning mundane tasks into challenges, like speed cleaning for 5 minutes, or use apps that track streaks such as Duolingo, Habitica or Streaks. You could even set a reward system for yourself, e.g., finish a task or earn a small treat.

Play Music That Gives You Chills- Listening to your favourite song can instantly spike dopamine. Upbeat, high-energy music works best.

Quick Read

Dopamine
The Reward Chemical

Hack It

Completing a task
Celebrating little wins
Self - care activities
Cold showers
Eat protein

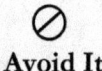

Avoid It

Excess social media scrolling
Junk food
Sugar spikes

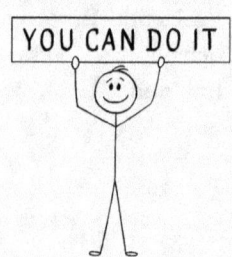

Dopamine spikes before the actual reward, so stretch out the excitement! **Increase Anticipation-**Look forward to something, such as booking a trip, planning a fun weekend, or saving a treat for later.

Newness Boosts Dopamine, so try novelty and learning a new skill, language, or hobby. You can also do this by changing your daily routine - try a new route to work, a new meal, or a new playlist.

Use the **flow State Trick.** This is where you fully immerse yourself in tasks like playing music, drawing, coding, or writing. Set a timer for 25 minutes and focus intensely - your brain rewards you with dopamine when you complete the session.

Practice Gratitude and Visualisation. Reflect on three things you are grateful for. This trains your brain to see rewards in your daily life. Visualising success before it happens tricks your brain into releasing dopamine as if you have already achieved it.

By intentionally using these tricks, you train your brain to produce dopamine naturally, keeping you motivated, focused, and in a better mood - without relying on unhealthy dopamine hits like excessive social media, sugar, or distractions.

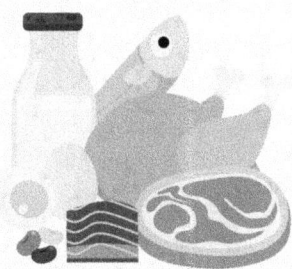

Along with intermittent fasting, you can also produce Dopamine by eating **protein-rich foods** that contain Tyrosine (a non-essential amino acid), including Eggs, Beef and Chicken, Salmon and Tuna, Cheese (especially Parmesan), Almonds and Peanuts, Whole Grains (Oats, Quinoa), Soy Products (Tofu, Tempeh, Edamame), and Bananas.

Things to Avoid
Suppose you stop bingeing dopamine triggers like social media, junk food, or excessive screen time; your brain resets and produces dopamine from more meaningful activities. So, take breaks from overstimulating content to feel real motivation again.

Oxytocin

Oxytocin, known as the "love hormone" or "bonding chemical," plays a crucial role in trust, connection, and emotional well-being. You can hack your brain into producing more oxytocin by engaging in simple, everyday activities that stimulate its release. Like **physical touch, which is** hugging someone for 20+ seconds. You can even hack this by touching yourself:

- **Hold Your Own Hands**
- Practice '**Havening**', cross your arms, and rub each arm from the shoulder down.
- Give yourself a **Massage-**rub your arms or shoulders, mimicking a human touch-or give yourself a **Butterfly Hug.** Full details on how to do this are overleaf.
- Or try a cuddle with a loved one, a pet, or even a warm blanket in bed.
- Physical Warmth, such as drinking a warm cup of tea or taking a warm bath, mimics the comfort of the human touch, as does wrapping yourself in a cosy blanket or wearing soft, comforting clothing.

Practice the "Soul Connection" Trick - simply making **Deep Eye Contact** for at least 30 seconds strengthens trust and connection. Even looking into your own eyes in the mirror while speaking kindly to yourself can help.

Give and Receive Acts of Kindness, i.e. do something thoughtful for someone without expecting anything in return and give a genuine compliment. This can boost oxytocin for both of you. Even small gestures, like smiling at a stranger, create an oxytocin spike.

Quick Read

Oxytocin
The Love Hormone

Hack It
Give a hug
Hold hands - even with yourself
Deep eye contact
Give kindness
Listen to moving music
Play with pets
Meditate
Laugh

Avoid It
Chronic Stress
Social Isolation
Lack of Physical Touch
Excessive Sleep Deprivation
Poor Diet
Excessive Alcohol and Drugs

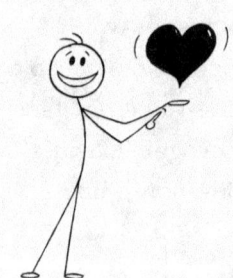

Listen to Music that Moves You and sing along. Group singing, like singing in a choir or with friends, supercharges oxytocin, as does playing an instrument, which stimulates oxytocin through self-expression. Other group activities like team sports, group workouts, or book clubs can also hack this. Even dancing or exercising with others helps boost social bonding.

Deep and Heartfelt Conversations can trigger the release of oxytocin by fostering emotional bonds. Even sending a genuine text message to someone you care about can create a positive effect. Also, **Genuine Laughter,** especially when shared with others, triggers the release of oxytocin. You can watch a funny movie, share jokes, or reminisce about a hilarious memory with a friend.

Interacting with pets, such as dogs and cats, or watching animal videos can release oxytocin. If you do not have a pet, consider visiting an animal shelter or observing wildlife in nature.

Meditate on Love and Gratitude. Close your eyes, focus on your heart, and think of someone you love. Practising loving-kindness meditation, which involves sending good thoughts to yourself and others, can also be beneficial.

Incorporating these habits into your daily routine can hack your brain into producing more oxytocin, leading to deeper connections, reduced stress, and a greater sense of well-being.

Things to avoid
Chronic stress and anxiety increase cortisol, which suppresses oxytocin release and reduces feelings of trust and connection. Social isolation and lack of meaningful interactions can significantly lower oxytocin levels, making it harder to experience emotional bonding - lack of physical touch. Excessive screen time and overuse of social media can create a false sense of connection while reducing real-life social bonding, which is essential for oxytocin production. Sleep deprivation negatively affects oxytocin regulation, leading to increased irritability and reduced emotional resilience. A diet low in essential nutrients, particularly magnesium, vitamin C, and omega-3 - 3 fatty acids, can impair oxytocin function. Excessive alcohol and drug use can also interfere with oxytocin receptors, reducing their effectiveness in promoting trust and emotional connection. To maintain healthy oxytocin levels, it is essential to prioritise face-to-face social interactions, physical touch, meaningful connections, proper sleep, and a nutrient-rich diet while minimising stress and digital distractions.

Serotonin

Serotonin, often called the "happiness chemical," is key to mood, well-being, and emotional stability. Unlike dopamine (which gives quick pleasure), serotonin promotes long-term happiness and calm.

The fastest natural serotonin boost is **Sunlight Exposure.** Simply go outside for 10 - 30 minutes of sunlight daily. Even on cloudy days, spending time outside signals your brain to release more serotonin. If sunlight is not available, try a light therapy lamp (great for winter months).

Move to Boost Mood - Cardio exercises like running, cycling, or brisk walking increase serotonin levels. Also, yoga and stretching - the key is consistency - just 10 - 15 minutes daily is enough to stimulate serotonin production.

Rewire your brain for happiness by **Practicing Gratitude** - write down three things you are grateful for daily. Or try the **"Mental Movie Trick"** - visualise a joyful moment and relive it.

Serotonin's secret ingredient is sleep! So, **get enough sleep.** Poor sleep lowers serotonin levels. Aim for 7 - 9 hours of quality sleep. Avoid screens one hour before bed (blue light disrupts serotonin and melatonin balance). Stick to a consistent sleep schedule to regulate your serotonin cycle.

Meditate and Breathe Deeply - Mindfulness increases serotonin by reducing stress hormones. Try box breathing: Inhale for 4 seconds, hold, and exhale for 6. Even 5 minutes of meditation or deep breathing can instantly boost serotonin levels.

Quick Read

Serotine
The Happiness Chemical

Hack It
Sunlight
Exercise
Gratitude
Get enough sleep
Meditate
Listen to music
Reduce stress

Avoid It
Chronic Stress and Overthinking
Poor Sleep Habits
Processed Sugar
Junk Food
Too Much Caffeine and Alcohol
Low Protein Diet
Vitamin D, B6, B12, Magnesium Deficiencies
No Sunlight
Lack of Exercise
Social Isolation

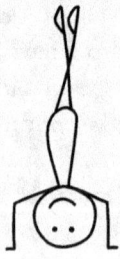

Have a 'Friendship Boost' Talking to a friend, family member, or loved one trigger serotonin. Even sending a text or voice note to someone you care about can improve your mood. Join social groups, attend events, or just smile more- small interactions activate serotonin pathways.

Engage in Meaningful Activities. Doing something that gives you a sense of purpose (helping others, creative hobbies, personal goals) naturally raises serotonin. Acts of kindness - like volunteering or giving compliments - boost serotonin in both you and the recipient!

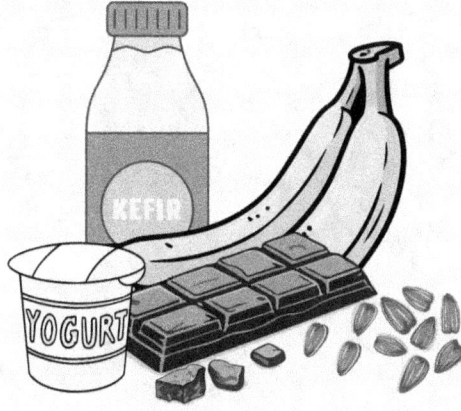

Eat Serotonin - Boosting Foods
Your brain needs tryptophan, an amino acid, to produce serotonin. Foods rich in tryptophan include:
- Bananas
- Dark chocolate
- Eggs
- Salmon
- Nuts, and seeds
- Fermented foods like yogurt kimchi, and kefir

Things to Avoid
Chronic stress and overthinking increase cortisol, suppressing serotonin production, while poor sleep habits disrupt serotonin's role in regulating melatonin, leading to mood imbalances. Excessive sugar and junk food cause temporary serotonin spikes followed by crashes, contributing to anxiety and irritability. In contrast, high caffeine intake can reduce serotonin receptor efficiency, making it harder to feel calm and focused. Alcohol and recreational drugs interfere with serotonin metabolism, leading to mood swings and long-term depletion. A low-protein diet deprives the body of tryptophan, an amino acid essential for serotonin production, and deficiencies in vitamins B6, B12, magnesium, and omega-3 - 3 fatty acids can further hinder serotonin synthesis. Lack of sunlight and low vitamin D levels also impair serotonin production. A sedentary lifestyle deprives the brain of the serotonin-boosting effects of exercise, and social isolation lowers oxytocin, which works alongside serotonin to regulate mood.

Melatonin

Melatonin is the sleep hormone responsible for regulating your circadian rhythm. It signals to your body when it is time to sleep and wake up. If you struggle with sleep or feel restless at night, you can hack your brain to produce more melatonin naturally by making simple lifestyle adjustments.

The biggest hack is to **Reduce Blue Light Exposure Before Bed.** The blue light emitted from screens (phones, TVs, and computers) suppresses melatonin production, tricking your brain into thinking it is still daytime. To prevent this, turn off screens at least an hour before bed. If you must use screens, enable Night Mode or wear blue-light-blocking glasses to minimise exposure. Use Red or Dim Lighting at night as bright white/blue lights suppress melatonin, while red, orange, or dim lighting promotes its release. Use salt lamps, red LED bulbs, or candlelight in the evening to help your brain wind down.

Morning exposure to natural light helps regulate melatonin production at night. Spending 10 - 30 minutes in sunlight (or near a bright window) within an hour of waking up helps reset your circadian rhythm, making it easier to fall asleep later. This natural light exposure signals to your body that it is daytime, helping regulate the sleep-wake cycle. **Stick to a consistent sleep schedule,** as going to bed and waking up simultaneously every day (even on weekends) helps train your body to release melatonin naturally at the right time. Irregular sleep patterns can confuse your brain, making melatonin production inconsistent. Keeping a stable routine

Quick Read

Melatonin
The Sleep Hormone

Hack It
Reduce Blue Light
Sunlight in the Morning
Consistent Sleep Schedule
Sleep in a dark cool room
Eat Melatonin rich food
Relax before bed with a
Warm Bath or Shower

Avoid It
Blue Light Exposure
Before Bed
Irregular Sleep Schedule
Artificial Light at Night
Caffeine in the Evening
Alcohol Before Bed
Eating Heavy Meals Late
at Night
Stress and High
Lack of Sunlight Exposure
During the Day
Overuse of Sleep
Medications
Noisy or Bright Sleep
Environment

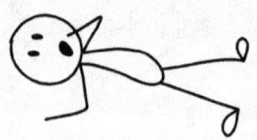

it reinforces your body's internal clock, ensuring better sleep quality. When you do go to bed, Keep Your Room Cool and Dark. Melatonin production increases in darkness, so making your room as dark as possible at bedtime is essential. Use blackout curtains or a sleep mask to block any excess light. Keeping your room cool (16 - 19°C or 60 - 67°F) also enhances melatonin release, as your body naturally lowers its temperature during sleep.

Try a Warm Bath or Shower Before Bed A hot shower or bath 1 - 2 hours before bed helps your body cool down faster, signalling melatonin release. Adding Epsom salts (magnesium) to a bath enhances relaxation and sleep quality. **Do Relaxing Activities Before Bed,** like reading, journaling, meditation and light stretching. Try deep breathing exercises (inhale for 4 seconds, hold for 4, and exhale for 6). Listening to calm music or white noise also encourages melatonin release.

Consider Natural Supplements (Only If Needed). Magnesium relaxes muscles and enhances melatonin production. L - Theanine, found in green tea, promotes relaxation without drowsiness. Or Melatonin Supplements - but only for short-term use.

By following these natural melatonin hacks, you will fall asleep faster, stay asleep longer, and wake up feeling more refreshed.

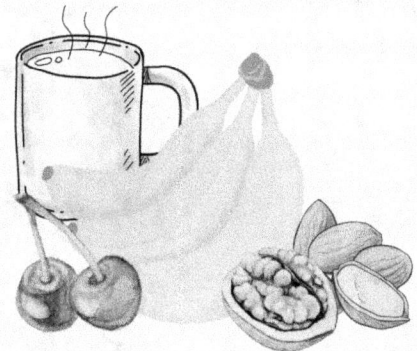

Eat Melatonin - Boosting Foods
Incorporating these foods into your diet can help support better sleep. Foods rich in melatonin include:
- Cherries
- Bananas
- Walnuts, almonds
- Oats and rice
- Turkey
- Warm Milk
- Herbal Tea chamomile, valerian root, and passionflower tea

Things to Avoid
Caffeine and Alcohol, as caffeine stays in your system for 6 - 8 hours and blocks melatonin production. Avoid it after 2 PM. Alcohol might make you drowsy, but it disrupts melatonin and REM sleep. Avoid screen and white light before bed

Glutamate

Glutamate is the brain's primary excitatory neurotransmitter, meaning it stimulates nerve cells and is essential for learning, memory, and overall brain function. It plays a crucial role in neuroplasticity, allowing the brain to form new connections and adapt to experiences. As one of the most abundant neurotransmitters, glutamate keeps the mind sharp, focused and engaged. However, an imbalance in glutamate levels can lead to neurological issues, including excess glutamate, which can overstimulate brain cells, contributing to anxiety, neurodegeneration, brain fog, and migraines. At the same time, too little glutamate can cause memory problems, fatigue, lack of motivation, and cognitive decline. Glutamate helps enhance learning, improve cognitive function, regulate mood, and support brain development when balanced. It also plays a vital role in motor control and coordination. Maintaining optimal glutamate levels is key to mental clarity, focus, and emotional well-being.

Boost it naturally by **engaging in new experiences,** such as learning a skill or new language or participating in regular exercise.

Eat Glutamate Boosting Foods
- Protein - rich foods
- Meat
- Fish
- Eggs
- Omega - 3 fatty acids
- Salmon
- Walnuts
- Flaxseeds

Quick Read

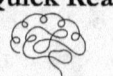

Glutamate
Neurotransmitter

Hack It
Reduce Blue Light
Sunlight in the Morning
Consistent Sleep Schedule
Sleep in a dark cool room
Eat Melatonin rich food
Relax before bed with a
Warm Bath or Shower

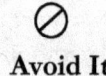

Avoid It

Too much MSG as this can give you excess glutamate which is a neurotoxin

Norepinephrine and Epinephrine

These neurotransmitters and hormones are crucial in the body's stress response, alertness, and energy regulation. They are produced in the adrenal glands and brain and help regulate the fight-or-flight response, which prepares the body to respond to danger or high-stress situations. Both are vital for mental and physical performance. They enhance focus, boost energy, regulate mood, and improve memory retention. In addition to their role in stress response, they help the body manage pain, inflammation, and metabolic function, making them essential for overall well-being.

Norepinephrine (Noradrenaline)

Norepinephrine is a neurotransmitter that acts primarily in the brain and nervous system, helping to enhance alertness, focus, and cognitive performance. It plays a key role in attention, motivation, and mood regulation, and imbalances in norepinephrine levels are often linked to anxiety, depression, and ADHD. This neurotransmitter also influences blood pressure and heart rate, ensuring the body remains energised and ready to respond to challenges.

Epinephrine, also known as adrenaline, functions as a hormone and a neurotransmitter. It is released in large amounts during stressful situations or emergencies, increasing heart rate, blood pressure, and energy levels. This surge in energy helps the body react quickly, whether in response to a physical threat or an intense emotional situation. While epinephrine is essential for survival, excessive levels can lead to chronic stress, anxiety, and high blood pressure.

Quick Read

Glutamate
Neurotransmitter

Hack It
Cold showers or ice baths
High - intensity workouts
Fasting
(short - term boosts catecholamines)
Adaptogens
(Rhodiola Rosea, ginseng)
Breathwork
(Wim Hof method, box breathing)

Avoid It
Chronic stress
(depletes norepinephrine reserves)

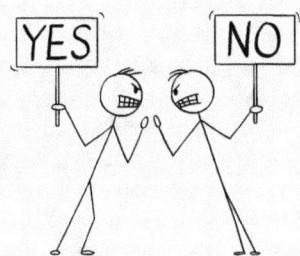

When norepinephrine and epinephrine levels are too high, individuals may experience anxiety, restlessness, high blood pressure, and difficulty sleeping. On the other hand, low levels of these neurotransmitters can lead to fatigue, depression, brain fog, and low motivation.

Hacking these naturally
This is more about keeping them in balance rather than boosting them. But there are still ways you can do this. It is important to engage in regular exercise, maintain a protein-rich diet (with tyrosine-rich foods like eggs, fish, and nuts), get quality sleep, and practise stress-reducing activities like meditation and deep breathing. Limiting caffeine, processed sugars, and chronic stress can also help keep these neurotransmitters in check.

By optimising norepinephrine and epinephrine levels, individuals can enhance their focus, energy, and emotional resilience, improving their mental and physical performance in daily life.

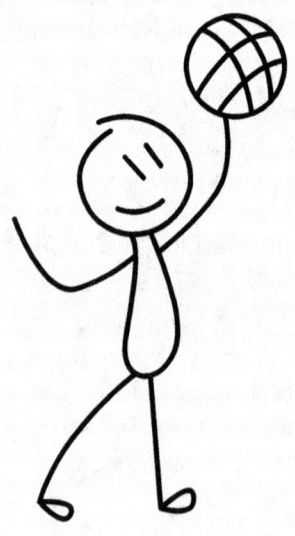

Acetylcholine (ACh)

This vital neurotransmitter is responsible for memory, learning, focus, muscle control, and overall brain function. It plays a key role in neuroplasticity, allowing the brain to form new connections and adapt to experiences. Found in both the central and peripheral nervous systems, acetylcholine helps regulate cognitive processes, attention, and muscle movement, including involuntary functions like heart rate and digestion.

An acetylcholine deficiency can lead to poor memory, brain fog, difficulty focusing, and muscle weakness, while excessive levels may cause muscle cramps, anxiety, and digestive issues.

Boost it naturally by **engaging in regular exercise**, **deep or new learning** (puzzles, reading and learning new things), and **meditation, which** can also support healthy acetylcholine function, enhancing mental clarity, memory, and overall cognitive performance. As can a power nap (20 minutes max)
Avoid: (depletes acetylcholine)

Consume choline-rich foods
- Eggs
- Fatty fish
- Beef liver
- Nuts and seeds

Quick Read

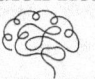

Acetylcholine
Neurotransmitter

Hack It
Exercise
New Learning
Puzzles
Reading
Meditation

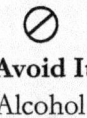

Avoid It
Alcohol
Smoking

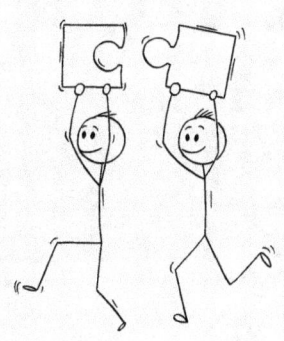

Endocannabinoids

These are naturally occurring neurotransmitters that help regulate mood, pain perception, appetite, memory, and overall balance within the body. They are part of the endocannabinoid system (ECS), which is crucial in maintaining homeostasis - keeping bodily functions stable and optimised. Endocannabinoids interact with cannabinoid receptors (CB1 and CB2) in the brain and nervous system, influencing stress response, immune function, and inflammation control.

Low levels of endocannabinoids can contribute to anxiety, chronic pain, poor sleep, and low mood, while balanced levels promote relaxation, emotional stability, and pain relief.

Natural ways to boost endocannabinoid production include **exercise, meditation, deep breathing, consuming omega-3-rich foods,** and **exposure to sunlight.**

Foods like dark chocolate, nuts, and flavonoids in fruits and vegetables also help support endocannabinoid function.

Balancing this system is essential for mental and physical well-being, stress management, and overall health.

Quick Read
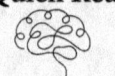
Glutamate
Neurotransmitter

Hack It
Dark chocolate
CBD oil
Exercise
Meditation
Deep breathing
Sexual activity

Avoid It
Chronic Stress
Poor Sleep Habits
Processed Foods
Lack of Omega - 3
Excessive Alcohol
Sedentary Lifestyle
Toxin Exposure
Overuse of Caffeine
and Stimulants

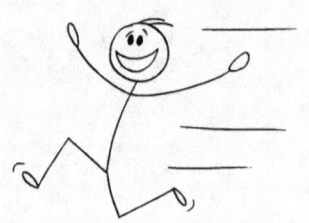

Endorphins

Endorphins are neurotransmitters that act as the body's natural painkillers and mood boosters. They are released in response to exercise, laughter, touch, and pleasurable activities, helping to reduce stress, relieve pain, and enhance overall well-being. Endorphins interact with opioid receptors in the brain, creating feelings of euphoria and relaxation, often referred to as a "runner's high" after intense physical activity.

Low endorphin levels can lead to increased stress, anxiety, low mood, and pain sensitivity, while higher levels contribute to happiness, emotional resilience, and reduced discomfort.

Engaging in **regular exercise, social interactions, laughter, listening to music,** and **consuming dark chocolate** or **spicy foods** can be highly effective ways to boost endorphin production naturally.

Maintaining balanced endorphin levels is crucial in mental health, stress management, and overall life satisfaction.

Quick Read

Glutamate
Neurotransmitter

Hack It
Exercise
(especially cardio and strength training)
Laughter
Spicy foods
Sunlight exposure
Listening to music that excites you

Avoid It
Chronic stress
(depletes norepinephrine reserves)

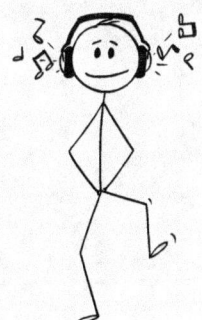

Cortisol

Cortisol is the body's primary stress hormone, produced by the adrenal glands in response to stress and energy demands. It regulates metabolism, immune function, blood pressure, and the sleep-wake cycle. As part of the fight-or-flight response, cortisol helps manage short-term stress by increasing alertness, focus, and energy.

However, when cortisol levels remain elevated for long periods, it can lead to chronic stress, anxiety, fatigue, and inflammation. High cortisol levels are associated with restlessness, weight gain, sleep disturbances, and sugar cravings, while low levels can cause fatigue, brain fog, dizziness, and low blood pressure.

To maintain healthy cortisol levels, it is important to manage stress, get **quality sleep**, **exercise moderately**, **eat a balanced diet**, and stay socially connected.

Proper cortisol regulation is essential for mental and physical well-being. It helps the body adapt to challenges while maintaining energy and balance.

Quick Read

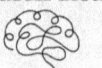

Cortisol
Neurotransmitter

Hack It
Daily meditation or breathwork
Quality sleep (7 - 9 hours)
Walking in nature
Journaling
Expressing emotions
Magnesium
Vitamin C supplementation
Laughter

Avoid It
Chronic Stress
Overworking
Sleep Deprivation
Excessive Caffeine Energy Drinks
Refined Sugars
Processed Foods
Lack of Physical Activity
Too Much High - Intensity Exercise
Skipping Meals
Extreme Dieting
Social Isolation Loneliness
Excessive Alcohol Consumption
Constant Exposure to Blue Light at Night

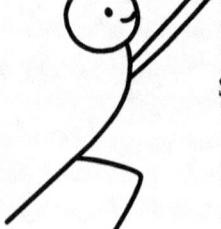

Histamine

Histamine is a neurotransmitter and immune system chemical that plays a key role in allergic reactions, digestion, sleep regulation, and brain function. It is involved in the body's immune response, triggering inflammation to fight infections or allergens, but it also acts as a neurotransmitter in the brain, supporting alertness, learning, and memory.

Histamine helps regulate the sleep-wake cycle, with higher levels promoting wakefulness and lower levels supporting sleep.

However, histamine imbalances can lead to various issues - high histamine levels may cause allergy symptoms, headaches, digestive problems, anxiety, and insomnia. In contrast, low levels can contribute to fatigue, brain fog, poor focus, and low motivation.

Consuming a nutrient-rich diet is essential for maintaining balanced histamine levels. This diet reduces exposure to allergens and processed foods, supports gut health, and manages stress.

Proper histamine regulation ensures a healthy immune system, optimal digestion, and balanced brain function, contributing to overall well-being.

Boost it naturally by **Regular fasting** (optimises histamine regulation), eat **Fermented food**s (kimchi, sauerkraut, kefir), **Avoid antihistamines** (they block alertness and focus)

Quick Read

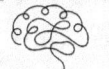

Histamine
Neurotransmitter

Hack It
To Increase
Eat Fermented foods like, Kimchi, Sauerkraut, and Kefir

Avoid It
To increase
Avoid antihistamines

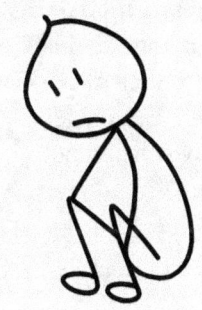

To reduce it, **avoid High-Histamine Foods**. Certain foods, including aged cheeses, cured meats, fermented foods, alcohol, vinegar, and smoked fish, naturally contain or trigger histamine release.

Processed and Preservative-Rich Foods - Artificial additives, flavour enhancers (like MSG), and preservatives can also increase histamine levels.

Excess Caffeine and Alcohol can block the enzyme DAO (Diamine Oxidase), which helps break down histamine, leading to a build-up.

Chronic Stress and Poor Sleep - High stress increases histamine release, while poor sleep disrupts histamine's role in the sleep-wake cycle. Certain Medications - Some painkillers (NSAIDs), antidepressants, and antibiotics can interfere with histamine breakdown.

Gut Imbalances and Poor Digestion - Damaged gut lining or low stomach acid can impair histamine regulation, leading to digestive discomfort and increased sensitivity.

Environmental Allergens and Toxins - Pollen, mould, dust mites, and chemical exposure can trigger excessive histamine release.

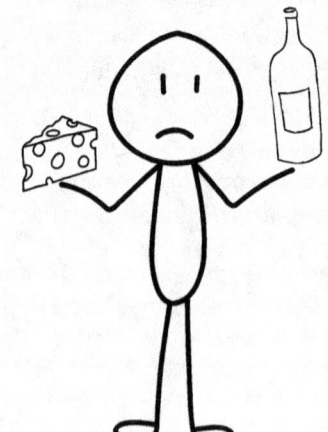

Quick Read

Histamine
Neurotransmitter

**Hack It
To Reduce**
Regular Fasting

**Avoid It
To reduce**
High - Histamine Foods - including aged cheeses, cured meats, fermented foods, alcohol, vinegar, and smoked fish.
Processed and Preservative - Rich Foods - Artificial additives, flavour enhancers (like MSG)
Excess Caffeine and Alcohol
Chronic Stress
Poor Sleep .
Some painkillers (NSAIDs), antidepressants, and antibiotics
Gut Imbalances and Poor Digestion .
Environmental Allergens and Toxins

Quick Fixes To Overcome Emotional Challenges

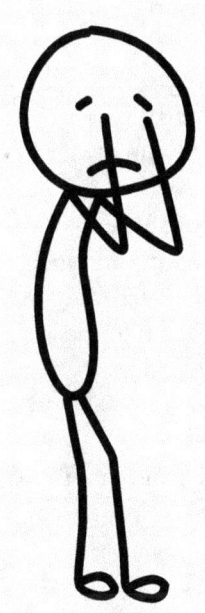

Each of these quick fixes helps to disrupt negative emotional cycles, giving you the space to regain control and respond more intentionally. It brings you back to balance and gets you back into the flow.

Deep Breathing (2 - Minute Reset)
Take a deep breath for four seconds, hold for four, and exhale for six. This will instantly calm your nervous system and help you regain control.

Name the Emotion (Awareness Shift)
Say aloud or write down your feelings: "I feel anxious," or "I feel frustrated." Acknowledging it reduces its power over you.

Change Your Posture (Physical Shift)
Stand up straight, roll your shoulders back, take a deep breath, or stretch. Your body affects your emotions more than you realise.

Cold Water Therapy (Instant Shock Reset)
Splash cold water on your face, take a cold shower, or hold an ice cube. This interrupts negative emotional loops.

Gratitude Shift (Perspective Flip)
When you are frustrated or sad, list three things you are grateful for in the moment. Gratitude rewires the brain for a more positive outlook.

Five Senses Grounding (Anxiety Reset)
Name five things you see, four you can touch, three you can hear, two you can smell, and one you can taste. This pulls you back into the present moment.

Power Playlist (Mood Booster)
Play a song that lifts your spirits and moves your body - music directly impacts your emotions.

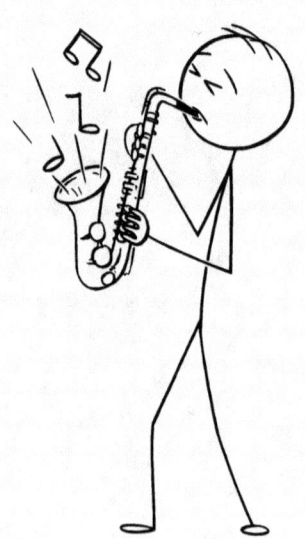

Laugh or Smile (Mood Booster)
Even faking a smile for 30 seconds can trick your brain into feeling better.

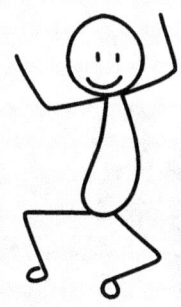

Journal it Out (Mind Dump)
Write down your thoughts without judgment. Getting them out of your head and onto paper helps you to process and release emotions.

Change Your Environment (Energy Shift)
Step outside, go for a walk, open a window, or switch rooms. A shift in scenery can help shift your mindset.

Affirmations (Rewire Your Thinking)
Repeat positive affirmations like "This is temporary," "I am in control of my emotions," or "I choose peace over worry."

Tapping (EFT - Emotional Freedom Technique)
Lightly tap pressure points (like the side of your hand, above your eyebrows, or under your collarbone) while affirming calming thoughts.

Mindful Distraction (Reset Focus)
Engage in an activity that shifts your focus - read, doodle, organise a small space, or do a simple puzzle.

Breathe and Delay Reaction (Pause Before Responding)
Before reacting emotionally, take three deep breaths and count to ten. A pause can prevent regretful decisions.

Talk to Someone (Verbal Release)
Sometimes, just venting to a trusted friend or therapist or even a voice note to yourself can bring clarity and relief.

About the author

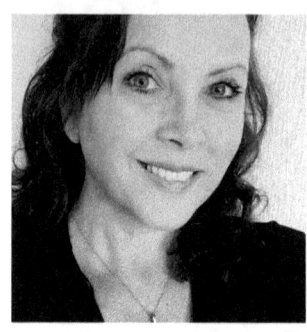

Teanna Taylor is a compassionate spiritual energy coach, meditation facilitator, and Energy Flows and Rainbow Breath Kids co-founder. With a heartfelt commitment to helping others tap into their inner strength, she also established Migraine Talk, a supportive platform for those navigating the challenges of chronic migraines.

Her story has resonated with many and has been featured in national and international magazines and newspapers. She has also shared her experiences on an international stage as a guest speaker at global pharmaceutical conferences and has facilitated meditation for over 14,000 people worldwide. Teanna has touched countless lives.

Teanna's journey took a transformative turn from a city career when she faced a minor stroke and endured a ten-year struggle with a debilitating migraine. Yes, one migraine 24/7 for a decade! She discovered the deep connection between mind, body, and energy through the many silent days and meditations. Combining scientific insights with ancient wisdom, she now empowers others through evidence-based techniques from neurology, psychology, quantum physics, and cherished spiritual traditions.

Residing in Whitstable, UK, with her four children, Teanna continues her heartfelt mission to help others heal, awaken, and unlock their highest potential. She understands many difficulties and is dedicated to guiding others toward wellness and self-discovery.

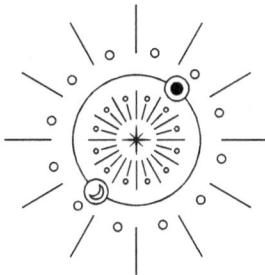

Also available by
Teanna Taylor

Cosmic Flow Spring Workbook
Sow The Seeds of Success

Cosmic Flow Summer Workbook
Cultivate Your Dreams

Cosmic Flow Autumn Workbook
Refine Your Vision

Cosmic Flow Winter Workbook
Align Inner Transformations

www.TeannaTaylor.com

www.ingramcontent.com/pod-product-compliance
Lightning Source LLC
Chambersburg PA
CBHW071154070526
44584CB00019B/2781